THE CRAFT OF LIFE

Earth Medicine is one of a collection of books written by Kenneth Meadows on the Craft of Life and how we, as individuals, can attune ourselves to Nature and the Earth and discover our own inner resources. Each book in the collection is a complete self-help manual in itself on an aspect of personal development towards a more fulfilling life.

For more than thirty years, **Kenneth Meadows** sought answers to some of life's most perplexing mysteries: Who am I? What am I? Why am I here? Where am I going? What is life's *purpose*? He explored the world's great religions and was offered *beliefs*. He considered the philosophies of great thinkers and gathered *opinions*. He examined the theories of materialistic science to find that most were based upon *assumptions*. His persistence brought him in touch with the simplicity of indigenous peoples whose wisdom had been passed on through oral traditions. He was directed to look not in the archives of learned institutions, but into the Book of Nature which reveals how the Universe *is* and that we humans are part of it and it is part of us. He found that by reconnecting with Nature we can make contact with our own Source and thereby find the answers we seek.

Kenneth, a Leeds University qualified teacher and former college lecturer and journalist, is internationally respected for his books on the application of shamanic principles to personal development and the extension of human potential. He has studied shamanic teachings directly under Native American, British, Scandinavian and other European shamans.

EARTH MEDICINE

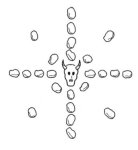

*Explore Your Individuality Through the
Native American Medicine Wheel*

Kenneth Meadows

CASTLE BOOKS

This edition published in 2002 by

CASTLE BOOKS

A division of Book Sales, Inc.

114 Northfield Avenue, Edison, NJ 08837

Published by arrangement with and permission of

Rider, an imprint of Ebury Press, Random House Group Ltd.

20 Vauxhall Bridge Road, London, SW1V 2SA

www.randomhouse.co.uk

Printed in the United States of America

ISBN: 0-7858-1491-4

Contents

Part One: The Philosophy

Part Two: The Analysis

Part Three: The Practice

Acknowledgements

My profound thanks and appreciation for making this book possible
go especially to:

Harley Swiftdeer, the Cherokee Metis-Medicine Chief, for giving me
my first practical experience of Medicine teachings.

Medicine Chief Silver Bear who has honoured me with much ancient
knowledge and commissioned me with the responsibility of passing
it on to others.

Wolf-Eagle for the benefit of his wisdom, guidance and understanding.

Tony Haggerstone and Leo Rutherford who shared some of my
experiences on the Medicine Way and whose advice was
invaluable.

My wife and life-long companion, Beryl, whose patience and understanding have sustained me throughout the task.

And to the Grandfathers and the Grandmothers. Ho.

Thank you, each and all. May you continue to touch the Earth with
beauty and bring healing to planet Earth.

Kenneth Meadows
(who was given the Medicine name 'Flying Horse')

Preface

*E*ARTH MEDICINE IS THE FIRST BOOK I COMPLETED IN WHAT HAS now become a collection of books which provide a distillation of ancient shamanic wisdom adapted to modern times and conditions and presenting a unique process of personal development which can change lives for the better.

Shamanics is the name I have given to this adaptation of shamanic principles to the practicalities of modern-day living. *Shamanics* is a word I coined to distinguish this process from the regurgitations of customs, rituals, and practices which have been taken from their tribal and historical context to form a feature of some representations of 'contemporary' shamanism, and which have little relevance to the challenges of everyday life in a modern society.

Earth Medicine is a method of exploring your own individuality and connecting with the potential powers that lie within you. The word *medicine* is used in its Native American sense to imply an empowerment that comes from within and which enables an individual to become more 'whole' or 'complete'. That empowerment connects him or her with the Earth and to the realm of physical reality. It is a principle based upon a shamanic understanding that Time itself has qualities which vary in accordance with the changing movement of the Earth as it orbits the Sun. These qualities are absorbed within our own energy-system at the moment of birth and so are inherent within ourselves. An understanding of *Earth Medicine* thus leads us not only to a fuller understanding of ourselves and others as personalities, but also enables us to come more into harmony with the benevolent forces of Nature which influence us from within as well as affecting us from without.

It helps us to recognize that the potentials we were born with are a part of our energy-system and that we can develop these potentials in order to fulfil the purpose of our lives for which they were given. *Earth Medicine* is an aid, too, to better human relationships for it helps in the understanding of others.

Since it was first published in 1989 by Element Books, *Earth Medicine* has been reprinted many times with translations into several foreign languages. The unsolicited complimentary letters I have received from so many appreciative readers in different countries are indications of the practical value of the principles and teachings it contains. This Rider edition is an updated version which draws on its past success in bettering the lives of those who read it.

Kenneth Meadows

Introduction

I HAVE CALLED THE SYSTEM OF SELF-DISCOVERY CONTAINED WITHIN these pages 'Earth Medicine' because it describes the nature of inner powers provided to each of us at birth through Earth energies prevalent at that time. Earth Medicine is derived from the 'hidden' teachings of the North American Indian Medicine Wheel and their correlation with the Taoist teachings of the East, and the shamanic wisdom of the ancient Caucasian peoples of Britain, northern Europe, and Scandinavia.

Earth Medicine is a method of personality profiling, based upon North American Indian Medicine Wheel principles which were part of the oral traditions of some tribes. Only now, with the Earth entering a critical New Age, which could become either a golden era of enlightened consciousness or an ecological and human disaster, is it necessary to make such teachings more generally available.

This book can show you:

- How to discover what you are, who you are, and what is a primary purpose of your life.

- How to release your creative energies and develop self-confidence through an appreciation and respect for this wonderful Earth that will put you in harmony with Nature and the environment.

- How to recognize subtle Earth influences and make use of them to bring you in tune with the pulse of the planet's time-energy.

- How to discover your own psychic sensors – your own totems – and make use of them to extend your awareness.

- How to obtain guidance and advice from your own Higher Self – your own 'Spirit' Self.

- How to compile monthly, weekly and daily 'readings' of the way the Earth energies are manifesting in your life and how they can be directed for your benefit.

Earth Medicine can free you from the impediment of assuming that you are the victim of circumstance or controlled by 'Fate', and help you to take responsibility for your own life.

Earth Medicine can not only help you to understand yourself and others, but bring about the kind of changes you want to happen in your life.

Quite literally, Earth Medicine can transform your life and give purpose and direction to your 'Earth Walk' and enable you to 'Walk in Beauty'.

PART ONE

The Philosophy

What *is* Earth Medicine?

YOUR EARTH WALK IS THE WAY YOU LIVE YOUR LIFE. IT IS THE WAY you express your personality. The way you live out your dreams. Your aspirations. Your hopes. Your fears.

Is your Earth Walk an aimless stroll, or a weary trudge? Does it show the flounce of impatience or the stiff step of anger? Or is it the brisk, determined stride of ambition which will let nothing stand in its way?

Whatever the mood of your Earth Walk, where are you on this Earth journey? Where are you situated now? Where have you come from? And where are you headed? Is life an exciting adventure, or just a bore? If you are bewildered through frustration and disappointment, if you are confused, is it not because you have no clear directions? You have been give no map of the territory, and you can see no signposts to guide you. You have no co-ordinates by which to plot your position, nor any chart on which to locate it. Is it, then, any wonder if life to you is an unsolvable puzzle?

Earth Medicine is a unique life science based upon North American Indian Medicine principles which had their origins in an even more ancient wisdom and which once lost, is now being regained. These principles were not confined to a particular tribe or group of tribes, but were the essence of a knowledge that impregnated them all.

This knowledge, though tempered in the American Indian mind, is structured here into a complete system which has been fashioned for modern times and adapted to the needs and circumstances of men and women living in a materialistic, consumer-orientated society that has lost its contact with Earth and with Nature.

The American Indian Medicine Wheel had many uses, including methods of self-knowledge and self-realization. Earth Medicine develops those methods and sets out to explain how the Soul puts on a garment of a physical body in order to experience matter and how, according to its position or perception point on the Wheel of Life, it connects with Earth influences and forces that can further its development through physical experience.

This system is not concerned with how the movement of the heavens might affect what happens to us in the future here on Earth, but with how our Earth connections may be used so that we can take *hold* of the present – in which our future is largely fashioned – and so assume responsibility for our own lives, and thereby attain mastery of our own destiny.

Perhaps before you picked up this book you had never heard of Earth Medicine. It has not been known because Medicine teachings themselves have been largely hidden within the oral traditions of American Indian Medicine men and protected by tribal shamans.

Before the period of great tribulation and suffering finally overwhelmed the much maligned and once proud and noble North American Indian people, elders representing principal tribes met together and determined that Medicine teachings were to be preserved by being conveyed orally down through the generations until it became possible for them to be practised fully again. The essence and spirit of the teachings were committed to their Sacred Fires, and to the spirits of the Elements with an assurance that they would be rekindled in another Age and at a time when the Earth itself would be in travail and suffering, and arise among people who were not of American Indian blood.

That time is now. Part of that knowledge is here in your hands and about to be communicated to you through the pages of this book.

However, before we can begin to grasp the basic principles, it is necessary to understand what the Medicine Wheel is.

To the North American Indian, 'medicine' meant more than a substance to restore health and vitality to a sick or maladjusted body. 'Medicine' was energy – a vital power or force that was inherent in Nature itself. A person's 'medicine' was their power – the expression of their own life-energy system. 'Medicine Wheel' meant a circle of generated energy – personal empowerment generated from a source that is within.

Basically, the Medicine Wheel is a physical, mental, emotional and spiritual structure that enables its users to attune themselves to Earth influences and forces and with the Source within themselves.

Some American Indians represented its circular structure with stones which were placed on the ground. Ancient stone circles in other parts of the world – and notably in Britain where there are the Rollright Stones on the borders of Oxfordshire and Warwickshire near the town of Chipping Norton, and Castlerigg in Cumbria – are larger examples and served similar, though not identical, purposes.

An advantage with the American Indian Medicine Wheel was its portability. A basic Medicine Wheel could be constructed by simply placing small stones in the form of a circle with spokes like a wheel. The four spokes, or arms, indicated paths to the centre which represented the Creator/Source or the Quintessence and which could also represent the self.

So it was a symbolic map or chart that could be set up anywhere.

The perimeter of the circle was marked by eight outer stones which represented powers in the Universe and within us and how they could be brought into harmonious balance. They served also as a reminder of the Law of Octaves – harmonic laws.

An inner circle of eight stones encompassed the 'Source' at the centre, and these represented inner and deeper realities.

The remaining eight stones formed the arms of a cross, two stones being placed in each of the four cardinal directions between the inner and outer circles. These four arms represented the Four Great Paths – Love and Trust in the South, Wisdom and Knowledge in the North, Introspection and Transformation in the West, and Illumination and Perception in the East.

American Indians sometimes used a buffalo skull to indicate the Source at the centre of the inner circle, and this was because the buffalo was particularly symbolic. In the old days, it was an animal that provided them with everything that was necessary for survival. Its flesh supplied food, its bones the material for making eating implements, tools and weapons. Parts of its body provided the means to fashion vessels for water and for cooking. Its hide was material for clothing and for covering their homes – the tipis – and its sinews the thread for sewing.

The human skull was regarded not just as a container for the brain – the human bio-computer – but as the seat of the consciousness. So a buffalo skull was seen as a representation of Wakan-Tanka – the Great Everything, the All That Is.

From this basic Medicine Wheel, an Earth Wheel can be constructed by adding a further 16 stones, or symbols, making a total of 40 to represent a universal web of power in which all things are connected.

Of these 16 additional stones, one can be placed in each of the four cardinal points to represent the Four Directional Powers, sometimes referred to as the Four Winds. The 12 stones formed the perimeter of the Medicine Wheel. Each represents a perception point and a segment of time in the Solar Cycle of the Year, and approximates to what we call a month.

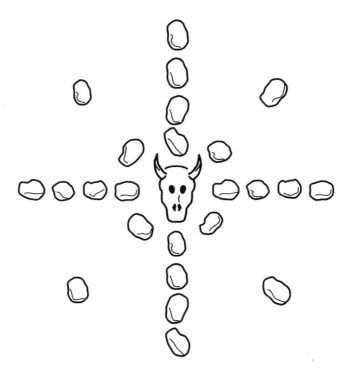

Figure 1. A basic Medicine Wheel of stones

The Medicine Wheel could be constructed of larger stones that made it suitable for numbers of people to participate, or of pebble-sized stones for use by an individual. Similarly, the Earth Wheel is adaptable and can be represented just as meaningfully by a simple drawing. It should be borne in mind that what is important is not the stones or masks themselves but the symbols the stones or marks on a piece of paper represent. Nor is it necessary to have a representation of a buffalo skull at the centre. Again, the important thing is to have in mind what the buffalo skull was there to indicate. In my view it is best to leave the centre empty as a reminder that the 'Void' is the invisible Source of Everything.

An Earth Wheel laid out in stones is shown in Figure 2.

A basic Medicine Wheel could be represented by simply drawing a cross within a circle, as in Figure 3, indicating the four cardinal directions.

Or taken a stage further, it could be drawn as a eight-spoked wheel and represented as in Figure 4 to include the four non-cardinal directions.

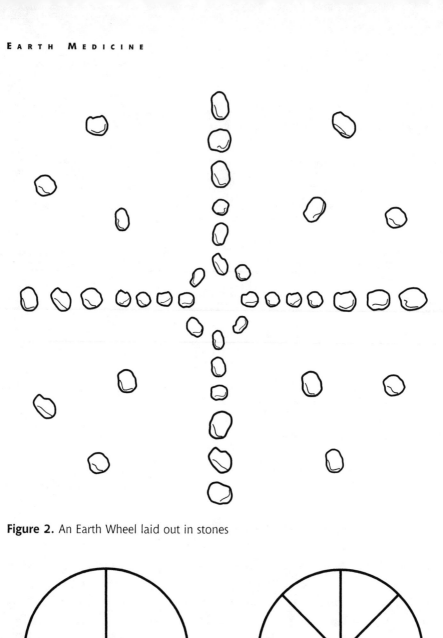

Figure 2. An Earth Wheel laid out in stones

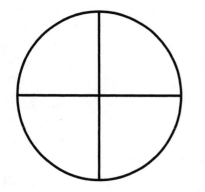

Figure 3. A basic Medicine Wheel of four cardinal directions

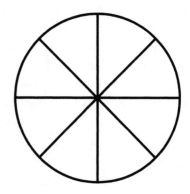

Figure 4. An eight-spoked Medicine Wheel including the non-cardinal directions

Essentially, Earth Medicine is a system of self-discovery. It does appear to have some similarities with Sun astrology since the twelve divisions correspond approximately to zodiac sign months, but it is not concerned with the movement of stars and planets and their possible influence on human affairs, nor does it involve complex calculations and such things as Rising Signs, aspects, transits and progressions. This is in no way intended as a criticism of Sun astrology. It is simply a different perspective calculated on the cyclic modulations of the Solstices and Equinoxes. Because of this connection with the seasons, the Birth totems for those born in the Southern hemisphere differ from those applicable in the Northern hemisphere. Guidelines are given later in this book for Southern hemisphere readers.

Sun astrology is founded on the principle, 'As Above, So Below', but our Earth Walk is influenced by another ancient concept – 'As Within, So Without' – and this is what is being emphasized in Earth Medicine.

There are three facets of Earth Medicine I should like to stress here at the outset:

First: Earth Medicine helps us to come to know and to understand *ourselves*. It is a means of discovering hidden potentials so that we can develop them and create for ourselves a more fulfilling life. It also helps us to understand others, so it is an aid to better human relations.

Second: Earth Medicine can help us to find meaning and purpose in our lives. It encourages us to accept responsibility for our own life and by so doing enhances personal freedom. So Earth Medicine champions true individual freedom which requires the constant companion of personal responsibility to walk alongside it.

Third: Earth Medicine helps us to free ourselves from being victims of circumstance, and instead to gain mastery of our own destiny. So Earth Medicine is an aid to taking *control* of our life.

Although Earth Medicine is based upon the American Indian Medicine Wheel, it embraces principles that are to be found in other cultures, too, for it shares vital aspects of the circular philosophy of ancient Britain and northern Europe, of Western esoteric traditions and of Eastern wisdom.

The reason is that all are derived from a common and very ancient source – the Wheel of Life and Circle of Power, which was the original

'Magik'* circle – and which is rooted in the distant past of all cultures and teachings and allegorized in the myths and legends of all peoples. It is so ancient that its origins became lost. Yet is has appeared throughout all ages and its presence is confirmed in the symbology imprinted on the artefacts that have withstood the corrosion of time.

This Wheel of Life is a Circle of Power – power over one's *own* life. That is why American Indians called it the *Medicine* Wheel, for in the terminology of the Indians, 'Medicine' meant 'power' and 'power' meant 'knowledge'. One might, therefore, define the Medicine Wheel as 'the Circle of Knowledge that gives power over one's life'.

This Circle of Knowledge and Power was the basis of the mystical teachings of ancient Egypt and Greece. The zodiac used in Sun astrology, the Cycle of the Year of Chinese astrology, the circular oracle of the I Ching, and the Ki oracle of the Japanese, all have their origins in it.

It has appeared as the mystical Cauldron of Cerridwin in ancient Britain, as the Round Table of the legendary King Arthur, as the Chalice of the Holy Grail, and as the Sacred Circle of pagans.

Whatever its symbolic representation in whatever age and in whatever culture, the Circle of Knowledge and Power – the Medicine Wheel – has served the purpose of a mirror. By looking into it one could see a reflection of the universe and come to an understanding of the 'mechanics' of natural laws and principles that energise and shape human lives.

In that reflection it was possible also to see the interdependence of all things and to discover one's relationship with all things, and thereby come into a greater understanding of the Totality of the 'Great Everything'. And it brought also a realization that what is seen and experienced in the world of objective reality outside ourselves, is itself but a reflection also of a subjective reality that is within, whether individually or collectively.

So the Circle of Knowledge and Power becomes a two-way mirror that can be looked into also as a *personal* mirror, a mirror of the 'little universe' that is the circle of awareness of the individual self. In it one can see the forces and energies that shape the individual self, and the characteristics and traits of the personality – the 'face' one presents to the world. And if we look into it deeply enough we may even catch a glimpse of the 'hidden' self, that

---

* Magik. This spelling is deliberate to make a distinction between the popular conception of magic associated with illusion and trickery, the supernatural use of the unseen forces of the universe under the control of mind, which is magick, and natural co-operation with Nature and the spiritual ecology.

'inner' self that is the True Self or Real Self and which some have called the soul or the Spirit Self.

That personal mirror is Earth Medicine.

When we look into the personal mirror of Earth Medicine we see a reflection of the core personality which the 'hidden' self has 'put on' for this lifetime like the clothing we wear. When we try on a new dress or hat, or a new shirt and suit, we use a mirror to see how we look, and to find out whether the clothes suit us. Earth Medicine is like that. It provides a means of checking over the personality 'garment' and the accessories that go with it – the qualities and attributes we have at our disposal in life – and the way we may appear to others.

When we look into an ordinary mirror, we see our blemishes as well as the features we like. Earth Medicine shows up our personality blemishes as well as our strengths so that we may do something about them too. And Earth Medicine indicates where to look to remove those blemishes that cause us so many problems in life.

So our weaknesses can become *opportunities* – opportunities to develop *new* strengths. For by recognizing our weaknesses rather than ignoring them or pretending they aren't there, we no longer need to make excuses for them. If we accept them positively, not as liabilities but as opportunities, we develop our individuality and strengthen our personality.

Our mistakes can be similarly recognized and accepted so that they become not excuses for remorse and self-pity over what might have been, but lessons that have been learned. For by recognizing a mistake and accepting responsibility for it, and making whatever amends we can for it, we convert it into a positive opportunity for our growth, and development into an individual who is better able to cope and who ultimately can be the master of any situation. That was part of the wisdom of the Medicine Wheel.

Earth Medicine thus develops an individual awareness of why we are what we are, and if we are dissatisfied with any aspect of our life, we can set about changing it so that we can become what the Real Self intended us to be.

At one time some Indians set about constructing a tangible reminder of the mirror-image of self they had discovered. For men, it was in the form of a shield – a personal shield.

This shield was never intended to be a physical protection against arrows or bullets, as most European settlers wrongly supposed, for it was far too fragile. Some were made from the tough hide of the buffalo or the bear, but others were constructed from softer skins, like those of the deer or the coyote. Each shield was painted with symbolic designs and decorated with feathers and fur, and each item represented in some way an aspect of the individual owner.

The shield thus identified its owner and described everything about him – not only who he was, but what he sought to be. Not just his skills and achievements, but his aims and aspirations. Not just his strengths, but his weaknesses and his fears.

A recognition of this helps us to understand an essential difference in attitude between the American Indian and those of us brought up in a materialistic society. The motivating factor in modern society is *getting* – achieving possession of *things* to make life more comfortable and pleasant or more enjoyable, or to confer status on the owner. The quest of life is directed by the question: 'What can I *have*?' the American Indian was motivated not by *getting* but by *be-ing*. His quest in life was motivated by the question, 'What should I *be*?'

If we are looking for something meaningful in our lives, perhaps there is a need for us to apply a little of the attitude of the American Indian.

The shield of a Native American woman was usually in the form of a belt which was worn around a dress. On it were woven symbolic designs with beads and quills, and these identified her in a similar way. Sometimes the designs were continued on the dress she wore.

Men and woman constructed their personal shield with great care because it was regarded not just as a physical object but as a reflection of the self.

This book provides you with all you need to construct your own personal shield, not out of hide and with paints and feathers and fur, but in the mind.

Your personal shield – your own mirror of self – will indicate the qualities you brought with you into this life, your inherent aptitudes, even some of the lessons you intended to learn in this life, and will help you to satisfy the quest to discover your own life's purpose.

I have indicated that Earth Medicine has certain similarities with Sun astrology. The interpretations of Sun astrology are arrived at through noting the positions of the Sun, Moon and planets in the circle of the zodiac at the time of one's birth, together with the degree of the ecliptic on the horizon (the Rising Sign or Ascendant). These are then related to each other, and interpreted in terms of the individual. Earth Medicine, however, is concerned with our connections with the Earth, with the elements, and with other forms of life which share the Earth environment with us – the mineral, plant and animal kingdoms. These connections act like wavelengths that enable us to tune in to the Whole and to understand the whole self. They also act like 'call signs' that enable us to contact the True Self within. Only two heavenly bodies figure in Earth Medicine – the Sun and the Moon – which are seen as regulating the ebb and flow of cosmic energies and forces into the aura of our own individual 'little universe'.

As in Sun Astrology, we enter life in a specific segment of the Earth Wheel. That becomes our starting-place or Sitting Place on the Wheel. It indicates how we came equipped to perceive the world we would find around us. But, of course, we do not stay the same. Circumstances, events, people, change us. We develop and evolve as individuals through the experience of living, just as our physical body changes and develops from that of an infant, to child, to youth, adult and eventual old age. Our physical body does not remain as it was. It changes to meet the needs of the phase or 'season' of life we are undergoing at the time. Nor does the self within remain in a fixed or static condition. It, too, 'evolves'. It moves.

The Medicine Wheel teaches that life is a process of change and development in the dimension of time. The future is largely fashioned in the present out of the fabric of the past. We each affect – and to a large extent determine – what we are going to become by what we do in the Here and Now. Our thinking and our actions, therefore, condition our future. It is not all mapped out for us in advance. We determine our own direction from the choices we make. We are not robots to some ethereal computer; we are the programmers. We program our own computer of self. Press the right psychological buttons and you change your thinking. Change the thinking and you change the attitude to the way things are done. Change the things that are done and you change the future.

So with Earth Medicine we are not stuck with things we can do nothing about. Earth Medicine encourages change. It helps us to get from where we are to where we want to be, and to become what we want to be.

Setting up the Circle

AMERICAN INDIAN TRADITIONS WERE BASED NOT ON A SET OF beliefs or on an interpretation of sacred writings, but on the knowledge of the pulsating rhythm of life that could be seen and sensed all around in the Book of Nature, in the chapters of the seasonal cycles, in the passages of the Sun and the Moon, and whose words could be found among the trees and plants and animals and birds.

The year was seen as a Great Circle with no actual 'beginning' or 'ending', and divided into periods of time – into seasons, related to the Sun, and into 'months', indicated by the Moon. The Great Circle was seen also to be divided into discrete sections of Earth influence that categorized the different ways in which the human being could broadly express itself on the Wheel of Life.

The Earth Wheel can be represented as a Web of Life and related to the natural cycles and to the cosmic energies that pulsate throughout all of Nature. But before we examine the construction of this web in detail, we need to understand how differently the Indian viewed the natural world as compared with ourselves.

We are conditioned in our thinking by the Age in which we live, which is one of scientific materialism. Scientific materialism is the science of matter – the investigation and explanation of matter and of the physical universe, in which all things are considered to have a physical origin.

Aboriginal peoples, like the ancients, were not so concerned with the science of matter, but rather with the science of spirit. Everything physical and material was, in essence, *manifested* spirit. The American Indian saw the universe and the whole of Nature as a *becoming* – a coming-into-being – whose essence was not material but spiritual. The physical environment and every part of it was derived and had its origins not from the material, but from the spiritual, and was in a state of continuous change.

Everything that came into being, or was coming into existence, had purpose, and everything that existed – whether it was mineral, plant, animal or human – was composed of *intelligent* energy. Nothing was ever destroyed, only changed. Matter was intelligent directed energy held together in harmonic synchronization. Everything was connected or linked by vibrations of light and colour and sound.

So when an American Indian shaman constructed a Circle which contained any representation of physical things, forces or energies, he was actually building a symbolic working model of how the Universe and the human being function. The two were not only similar, but integral. We need to bear this concept in mind as we examine how the Earth Wheel or Web is brought into being.

The Earth Wheel is based upon the natural cycle of the year and the four seasons as the Earth orbits the Sun, and which governs the environment in which we find ourselves in this physical dimension of existence. And this demonstrates another important concept:

Most of us have been educated to think mechanistically. That is, we think 'logically' in straight lines, assuming that everything has a beginning and an ending. But neither the American Indian nor the ancient peoples thought that way.

The Indian observed that there were no straight lines in Nature. The Sun and the Moon were round, and so was the Earth. The rising and the setting of the Sun was a circular motion. The Moon traced a circular pattern in the sky. Birds built their nests in circles. Animals marked their territories in circles. The growth pattern of trees and rocks was circular. Many Indians lived in circular homes called tipis, and native communities were set up around a circle because the whole of Nature expressed itself in circular patterns. Only the white man, it seemed, thought of everything in straight lines.

The seasonal movement of the Sun and the monthly cycle of the Moon, which mainly condition our Earth environment and energies, reflect this important concept, too. So let us see how the Earth Wheel or Web comes into being:

First, there is the circle itself.

We start with a circle because a circle is a *container*. To the Indian, the circle represented what we may call the universe. It was a totality of space. But it also represented the individual and everything around the individual – so we could call it also the individual's own personal space, or personal universe.

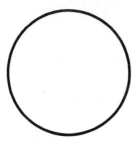

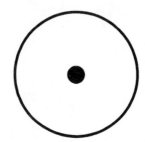

Figure 5. The 'container' of space

Figure 6. The 'centre' around which is the space of existence

If we put a dot in the centre we have a very ancient symbol for the Infinite becoming finite, a representation of the cosmic centre at the heart of infinity, of the Source of Light and of Life, of the Source at the centre of the universe. But it is also a symbol of our own individual consciousness coming into manifestation in the centre of our own personal universe.

Now try to imagine the circle not as a flat, two-dimensional image on the surface of the page, but as multidimensional, extending all around you in every direction so that the centre of the circle is the centre of a sphere or globe which extends upwards and downwards as well as outwards.

The circle we have drawn on paper might be compared with slicing that sphere through its equator. Imagine yourself standing through that dot in the centre, so there is an 'up' above your head, a 'down' beneath your feet, a direction in front of you and behind you, and to your left and to your right (see Figure 7).

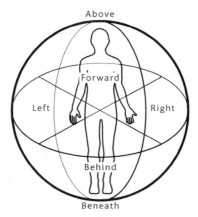

Figure 7. Our sense of direction within space

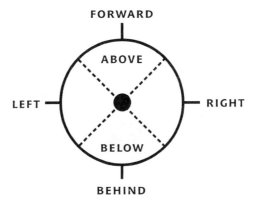

Figure 8. Our circle of Awareness

So here you are in the centre of your own universe in which you are to experience conscious existence on the plane of physical reality. But you have nothing to relate to. You have only a position in space. You require reference points and co-ordinates in Time to enable you to know where you are and to be conscious of movement from one place to another.

In our physical environment, time can be 'marked' by the boundaries of darkness and light in the daily cycle and by the solstices of the shortest day and the longest day in the yearly cycle.

We can 'plot' these on the circle. By drawing our circle of awareness on a piece of paper we can divide it into four directions, each occupying 90 degrees – Forward, Behind, Left and Right (see Figure 8).

By placing the shortest day or the Winter Solstice (22 December in the Northern hemisphere) at the 'beginning' of the 'Forward' portion – that is, assuming a sunwise or clockwise movement – and the longest day or Summer Solstice (around 21 June in the Northern hemisphere) directly opposite at the 'start' of the 'Behind' portion, we have established two directional positions and polarities.

For general purposes, the Medicine Wheel is cast with the north in front and the south behind and since we are viewing this representation on a flat, two-dimensional plane, relate yourself to the drawing as if you are facing north from a position in the centre (see Figure 7).

With a single line, we have not only divided the circle and separated night from day, and indicated the respective positions of midsummer and midwinter, but we have dissected space and established a position in time. We have established two sets of time-periods that enable us to 'ground' our

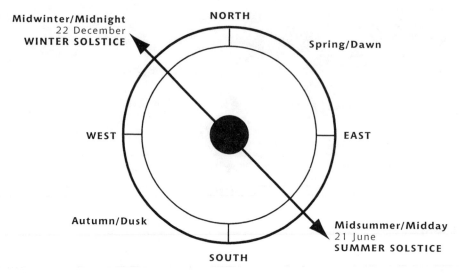

Figure 9. The Solstice co-ordinates

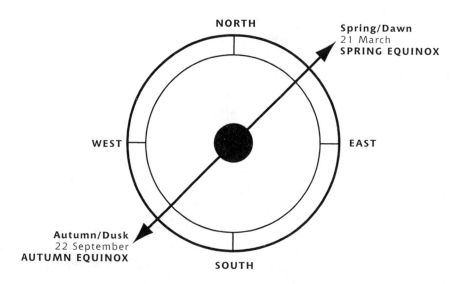

Figure 10. The Equinox co-ordinates

concept and to place it in the world of practical reality – midnight and midday, midwinter and midsummer.

There are two other reference points we can establish. These are dawn and dusk, and in the yearly cycle these correspond to the days when the period of night and the period of day are of equal length – the Spring and Autumn Equinoxes. In the yearly cycle these occur exactly half-way between

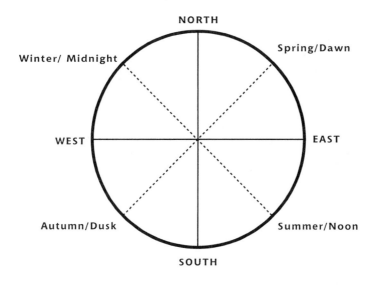

Figure 11. The eight-spoked Wheel of Time

the Winter and Summer Solstices and provide us, therefore, with a north-east and south-west axis and two more firm dates to help us (see Figure 10).

By putting all this together we have an eight-spoked wheel, or a hub in the centre of a circle that is connected to the perimeter by eight arms. Four of these arms or spokes indicate the cardinal directions of north (ahead) and south (behind), and east (right) and west (left), and the other four provide the non-cardinal 'time' markers of dawn and spring (north-east), noon and summer (south-east), dusk and autumn (south-west) and midnight and midwinter (north-west) (see Figure 11).

The eight-spoked wheel was a symbol that embraced a number of ancient teachings. One was that every living thing contains four primary forces in perfect balance. These four primary forces are unique, intelligent expressions of the Source of existence.

It was composed of an encircled cross which indicated the activity of the binding force and the life-force, and a cross within a circle which indicated electromagnetic force and vibratory force. The vibratory force found expression in laws, the electromagnetic force in light, the binding force in

Love and the Life-force in life. So the universe is constructed on four great creative principles – Light, Life,
Love and Law which could be represented in an eight-
armed cross which indicated the dual nature of each, and
this was placed within the Circle of Existence. Our simple
construction has thus assumed profound meaning based
upon just two fundamental principles – Love and Harmony.

 This construction may also be said to be solar-orientated
because it follows the cycle of the day and night and of the
seasons of the year, each of which are dependent on the
Earth's orbit around the Sun. We know that the Earth's tilt
varies up to $23\frac{1}{2}$ degrees either way of its axis, so the various areas of the
surface are exposed to a higher density of the Sun's rays at certain times
during the Earth's orbit, and it is this which causes the seasons.

The natural cycle of the year is thus inseparably linked with the intelligent expressions of the Creative Source and is therefore a vital key to their
understanding.

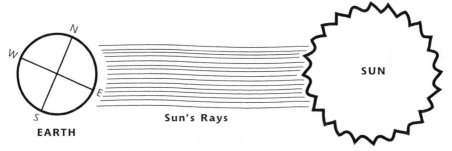

Figure 12. Summer in the Northern hemisphere. Northern hemisphere tilted
towards the Sun.

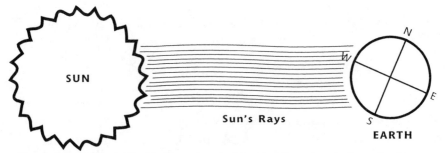

Figure 13. Winter in the Northern hemisphere. Northern hemisphere tilted away
from the Sun.

At the Summer Solstice more of the Northern hemisphere is in direct contact with the Sun's rays than at the Winter Solstice. In the summer, more intensive solar rays are received than in winter, and this is an important principle to bear in mind when considering the effect of the hidden forces of Nature, not only on the environment, but on ourselves (see Figures 12 and 13).

The Sun

Before we proceed further in the construction of the Earth Wheel, let us consider something of the significance of the Sun. The Sun is a mighty star at the centre of our universe, around which our Earth and all the planets revolve. So awesome is its power that it holds these vast bodies in place and in precise individual orbits, and it powers their travelling at tremendous speeds of thousands of miles a second.

The Sun is our source of light. So it is our Light-giver. It is our source of life, for no life on Earth could exist without it. So it is also our Life-generator and Life-maintainer – the great motivating and animating force of the solar system.

This solar force that penetrates all things, this thrusting primary energy source, was referred to in Amerindian cosmology as 'Grandfather Sun'. Grandfather Sun was a symbolic personification, not of the *physical* Sun itself, but of the Absolute Source that exists beyond the physical manifestation.

The ancients taught, too, that the Sun was symbolic also of the Real Self or True Self 'within' that I mentioned earlier, which is at the centre of our own being and is the 'Sun' of our own individual 'little' solar system.

The Sun was considered to have four phases:

Dawn is the rising Sun, the bringer of life with the promise of day.

Noon is the midday Sun, reaching its full power and bestowing life on all, energizing all activity, and powering all that grows.

Dusk is the setting of the Sun at the end of the day, and signals the time of rest, refreshment and renewal.

Night is when the Sun appears to have died and to have vanished into oblivion, but with the promise of its rising anew with each new dawn.

Although the seasons themselves actually *merge* into one another, each possesses special qualities of its own:

Spring is the time of abundant energy and vigour, and of a striving for growth.

Summer is the time for flowering as growth is achieved.

Autumn is the time of harvesting and gathering in and when life begins to withdraw into the seed.

Winter is the time when withdrawal is complete and life lies dormant in the seed waiting to be awakened when warmth returns with the Sun in spring and the cycle begins again.

This seasonal cycle was likened to human life and to the 'seasons' of our years.

Spring represents the years from birth and infancy through *childhood*.

Summer represents the years of youth and the growing into *adulthood*.

Autumn represents the years of *maturity* and of gathering in the fruits of one's endeavours.

Winter represents the years of physical decline but the development of *wisdom* which has been gained from the lessons of the life-experience. It also includes old age and the transition of death before the cycle begins again.

The Moon

Our environment on the Earth and the circle we are constructing is affected by another cyclic power – the Moon. The Moon has an immense effect on the Earth and on the bodies of all living things, including ourselves, during its orbit of approximately 29 days round the Earth. This cycle is the origin of the month (a word which means 'moon').

The Moon's magnetic gravitational power, combined with the movement of the Earth, causes the rise and fall of vast oceans and the fluctuation of the tides. It influences the flow of sap in trees and plants and of body fluids, including the rhythm of the blood, the female menstrual and gestation cycles, and the brain itself.

There are three principal cycles of the Moon;

The *first* is the orbit of the Moon around the Earth which takes approximately 29 days. In this cycle the Moon is seen first as a narrow crescent of the New Moon which waxes to Full and then wanes to a thin crescent before is disappears and becomes Dark, then appears again for the next cycle as the New Moon.

The *second* cycle is in the variation of its distance from the Earth as observed by the size of its appearance. This is due to the Moon following an elliptical orbit around the Earth. When the Moon appears at its largest it is closest to the Earth and its power is felt to be more than 25 per cent stronger than when it is at its smallest and its furthest distance from the Earth.

The *third* cycle is in the variation of its height in the sky. This is because the Moon's orbit is not parallel with the Earth's Equator, so it appears to 'wobble' and be higher in the sky at some times than at others.

Each of these cycles affects the power that the Moon exerts on the Earth and on all living things, including ourselves. Whereas the Sun can be used to symbolize the essential self, and the Earth to represent the physical body and the senses the self uses as a vehicle, the Moon symbolizes the reactions and responses between the two.

The new Moon marks the start of each lunation cycle which begins when the Moon is invisible and in the same direction as the Sun in the sky, and reaches its climax as the Full Moon which is half-way through the cycle. Each cycle takes approximately 29 days, so there are 12–13 cycles in a Solar Year.

The lunation cycle, or cycle of phases, it not the same as the zodiacal cycle of approximately $27^1/_2$ days. The Moon's phase is different at corresponding times in any solar or Earth month calendar, but its influence must be considered at all times.

So, in addition to the seasonal quarters, we have now established another important influence on us – the Moon.

The Twelve Segments

We can divide each seasonal quarter into three, and we then have a total of twelve sections, or divisions, or segments within our Earth Wheel which now takes on a pattern that relates to the organizational structure of Nature (see Figure 14).

Do keep in mind that the Wheel we have now been constructing is only a *representation*. It is a classification system. It is a symbolic structure –

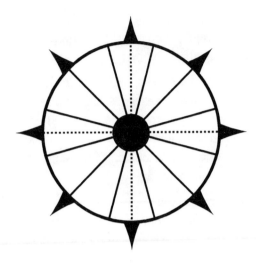

Figure 14. The twelve segments of the Earth Wheel within the eight Directions

a chart, or model with which to work in our quest for self-discovery. It is a map to help up to find our way and, like a map, it is not the territory itself.

In ancient wisdom, 12 was the number of 'measurement'. It was also the number of 'organisation'. In other words, it was the number for the arrangement into a systematic whole. And here the Earth Wheel presents us with twelve time periods which, as we shall see, are also twelve ways of categorizing personality. They indicate twelve different personality 'masks', twelve different 'faces', twelve kinds of personality the self can 'put on' and present to the world and with which to experience the world.

The ancients ascertained that there were twelve broad categories of perceiving and experiencing the physical dimension on the Wheel of Life – twelve Personality 'masks', twelve broad Earth 'influences'. There was a thirteenth influence, or Moon, an influence that was the sum total of the other twelve, but it was not included on the Wheel. It was represented by its very omission! That may seem like a conundrum, but let me explain.

The thirteenth influence is not excluded for any superstitious motive. There is nothing ominous or sinister or 'unlucky' about the number 13 in ancient wisdom. Thirteen often symbolizes *transition* – a dramatic change of movement from one level to another.

The thirteenth influence is not plotted on the Earth Wheel because it represents 'time out of time' – a period of transition which is experienced *outside* the circle of our existence on the physical and material plane. It cannot be portioned because it exists on another dimension outside the boundaries of matter and the limitations of time. It cannot be 'positioned' because transition – what we call 'death' – does not necessarily come to all people in old age. It occurs to different people at different ages – sometimes in old age, but sometimes in their prime, sometimes in youth, and even in childhood or infancy. The thirteenth influence cannot, therefore, be plotted but may be considered to be represented by the space at the centre of the circle.

Although it is not plotted, it is 'there' to represent when the conscious entity leaves the circle of the material realm and vanishes into the 'invisible' on a curve of a spiral that transfers it to another dimension. It re-enters the circle in due course to begin again another cycle of physical existence to put on, possibly, a different personality mask in a process we call reincarnation. The cycle of birth, growth, maturity, death, withdrawal and rebirth applied to the human being and was demonstrated throughout all Nature.

American Indians understood the human condition and purpose through a comprehension of the changes taking place *on Earth* – in the movements of the seasons and the moons and in Nature all around. It was recognized that there was a dynamic interaction between an active and passive duality that existed in all things. There was an active, conceptual and masculine polarity which was associated with light and the Sun, and there was a passive, receptive, feminine polarity, the reflected light that was associated with the Moon. The thrusting, positive, masculine principle was constantly seeking union with the receptive, 'negative', feminine principle which was constantly seeking to be possessed by its complementary opposite. These activities had an enormous effect on the Earth and thus on those living on her.

The ancient oriental philosophers expressed a similar idea in the Tai Chi mandala – a symbol which expressed the duality which came out of the Ultimate Reality that existed before the universe began. The Tai Chi represented the beginning of existence when the positive, masculine *yang* and the receptive, feminine *yin* came into being to become the ever-present life-force in all things that come into existence and which are the polarities that provide the rhythm and movement of constant change, for the yang and yin each contained within it the seed of its polar opposite.

The yang and yin principles were not regarded by ancient peoples as antagonistic opposites like the God and Satan concept of monotheistic religions. They were looked upon as complementaries, as co-equal and co-operating partners in the process of continuous Creation.

In ancient British and northern European and other traditions, these same forces were referred to as the god and goddess, and in ancient Egypt as Osiris and Isis. However, they are the personifications of spiritual principles and a means of helping the human mind to relate to them.

Since the yang and yin concept has become popularized in the West and these terms are 'neutral' and therefore less likely to be associated with a particular religion or belief system, I shall make use of them in this book in endeavouring to explain the basic principles of Earth Medicine.

These two interacting forces can be understood through the solar cycle of activity in which the Sun (yang) is used to represent the Source of Life, and through the lunar cycle of activity in which the Moon (yin) is used to represent the Sustainer of Life. The Sun can represent the source of creative energy available to an individual, and the Moon the power that gives form to that energy and makes an actuality of what was before just a potential. The Sun can also be related to *conscious* activity (yang) and the Moon to *subconscious* activity (yin).

In relation to Sun and Moon, the Earth is both yang and yin, and reacts to them variously. We are affected by Sun, Moon and Earth, and by their reactions to each other, and are ourselves subject to yang and yin influences.

This yang and yin principle thus affects us fundamentally and saturates our entire being. For instance, man might be described as vigorous and firm and therefore yang, while woman might be described as passive and gentle and therefore yin. We are each, whether male or female, a complexity of these two dynamic forces and we are expressing them in various ways. So whether we are male or female, yang or yin predominates in aspects of our characters and in our attitude. For instance, a yang person likes to take things apart and analyse them to see how they work. A yin person likes to bring things together and get them to harmonize. A yang person is striving and enterprising and involved in practical activity. A yin person is introspective and individualistic and concerned more with personal development. A

Figure 15. The light portion of the circle represents the positive creative force (yang), the dark portion the receptive and nurturing force (yin), and the dots in the centre the seeds of change which produce polar reversal and periodicity. This constant movement in the striving for union generates the creative energy that manifests in new life and in all forms.

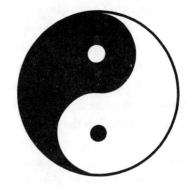

yang person is involved in practical work. A yin person is more concerned with ideas.

In a 'working' model of the Medicine Wheel we can relate yang to that which is 'above' (sky) and yin to that which is 'below' (Earth) as viewed from a position in the centre of the Circle.

It is from the cosmic duality principle of the yang and yin that the Four Primary powers came into existence and found expression in what the Indian described as the Four Winds. And it is from this same principle that the Four Elements, from which all physical matter derives, also came into being. As we shall discover later in this book each of the Four Winds and each of the Four Elements has characteristics and qualities which affect all living things whether they be human, animal, plant or mineral. And each is associated also with one of the four seasons of the year.

Each directional power affects the three sections of its own quarter – or three segments of Earth influence time – and its qualities are reflected in people born during those periods.

Just as we are affected by light from the Sun and the degree of its intensity and seasonal changes, so the light energy of the Moon has an influence. Moonlight is reflected sunlight, and the power of that sunlight is suffused and modified. The intensity of Moonlight varies greatly throughout a lunar month depending on the particular phase of the Moon and this also has relevance to the influence of the directional power.

It must be stressed that the stage of the Moon at a particular time must always be considered in conjunction with the Earth influence time as it is essential to work with the ebb and flow of the lunar currents which powerfully 'drive' the Earth influences.

There are four *stages* of the Moon, which are the varying degrees of light that it reflects from the Sun in its journey counterclockwise around the Earth – from the Dark of the Moon when its surface is completely dark, to the Full Moon when its surface is fully lit, and back again to fully dark.

The *first stage* is when the Moon is not visible because it is rising in almost the same direction as the Sun. At the end of this stage, a thin crescent can be seen as the Moon follows the Sun on the western horizon. The Dark of the Moon lasts for four days and is followed by the New Moon as the thin crescent appears. Applying the yang-yin principles this stage would be yin ▬ ▬ .

The *second stage* is when the Moon and the Sun are at right angles to each other. The Moon can be seen in the west during the first half of the night. During this stage the Moon appears to be getting fatter, so this is the stage of the Waxing Moon. This stage lasts for eleven days and is yin to yang **━ ━** .

The *third stage* is when the Moon and the Sun are opposite each other and the surface of the Moon is fully lit. This stage is called the Full Moon and lasts for three days with the night of the Full Moon falling on the third day. This is yang **━━** .

The fourth stage is when the Sun and Moon are again at right angles to each other, and the Moon is seen in the Eastern sky. As this stage progresses the Moon appears to be getting thinner and reduces to a narrow crescent. This stage lasts for eleven days and is yang to yin **━ ━** .

Waxing Moon	**Spring**	**Indicated**	**The Time**
The 'face' of the *Maiden*	Starts with the Spring Equinox on 21 March	Inception and expansion	of preparation
Full Moon	**Summer**	**Indicated**	**The Time**
The 'face' of the Mature Woman; *Mother*	Peaks with the Summer Solstice around 21 June	Maturity and fulfilment	of 'outer' development of the personality and the individuality
Waning Moon	**Autumn**	**Indicated**	**The Time**
The 'face' of the wise old lady; *Grandmother*	Starts with the Autumn Equinox on 22 September	The teaching or giving out of acquired wisdom	of 'inner' development
Dark Moon	**Winter**	**Indicated**	**The Time**
The 'face' of the aged woman; *Hag*	Troughs at the Winter Solstice around 22 Dec	The potential; rest; repose; reincarnation	of preparation for new beginnings

The Form of Human Expression

The Moon can also be seen as representing the power that gives form to the individualized spirit (represented by the Sun) in the dimension of matter (represented by the Earth). The Moon is also related to the human personality while the Sun is related to the individuality of the spiritual 'self'.

The twelve divisions of the Earth Wheel also indicate the twelve stages of expression and development on the 'evolutionary' path of the soul. This path was symbolized in various cultures and in pre-Christian times by the four faces of the Moon Goddess – Maiden, Mother, Grandmother, Hag (see chart opposite).

The seasonal path thus follows a cycle from birth, through expansion and growth to maturity and fulfilment and the acquisition of wisdom, and then through decline of the physical but expansion of the spiritual, to rest and transition. During the period of rest and transition – represented by the nights when the face of the Moon is hidden – the creative act takes place and the rejuvenation that precedes new life with a New Moon. And so the cycle is repeated – Moon, Sun, Earth and us all dancing the same tune.

We have therefore, an ever-turning Wheel of Life which is fashioned in Time's workshop. Since there are twelve equally balanced segments, we can allocate a roughly equivalent portion of time to each, and since the Spring Equinox provides us with a 'fixed' entry point, we can begin our calculations there. The four seasonal 'arms' provide us with firm check-points.

Our Earth Wheel can now be give a web-like appearance as in Figure 16.

Thus, we have developed a simple 'wheel' into a basic web-like construction which more clearly indicates that all things that exist within it are interconnected through a fine network of strands or threads. We shall see later how this develops into a more complex structure.

This web-like arrangement can be related to all things in existence on Earth, including ourselves. And since existence is not merely physical and material but is experienced on emotional, mental and spiritual levels, our Web can also be a chart to other levels of consciousness, whether 'above' or 'below' the frequency of our normal range of conscious awareness.

A web-like structure also serves as a reminder that all things are part of a greater whole and connected and interrelated through the life-essence or 'spirit' that is within all things that have existence and which is at the very source of their identity and individuality.

This spirit or energy-force is within every human being, within all animals, birds and creatures that swim and crawl, within plants and trees,

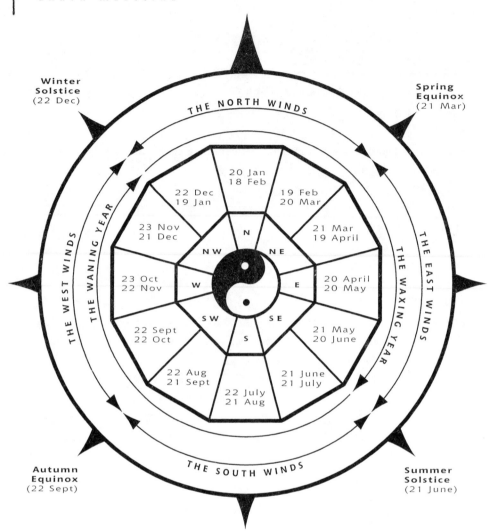

Figure 16. The Earth Web and its relationship with the solar year

and within rocks and stones and minerals. It is even within the very elements themselves – within Water and Fire and Earth and even Air, for it is in the very winds that freshen and vitalize us and keep us 'alive'.

Our basic Web of twelve segments contains and absorbs within it the eight-spoked 'Wheel' which, as we shall see, is a vital 'component' in the way the Web functions. In this Web the flow of energy or power moves from the unseen – the non-physical – to the seen, to that which appears; from the realm of that which is not yet manifest to the realm of appearances; from what some American Indians called the 'Nagual' to the 'Tonal', to the everyday world of 'ordinary' existence.

The Eight Directions

THE TWELVE SEGMENTS OF THE EARTH WEB, LIKE THE ZODIAC AND the Wheel of the Year of Chinese astrology, are an extension of an earlier and more ancient system in which there were only *eight* divisions or directions – north, north-east, east, south-east, south, south-west, west and north-west (see Figure 17).

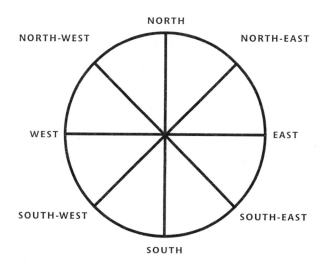

Figure 17.

The Eight-Directions 'Wheel' is a structure that has been used throughout history and by all cultures, and this is evident from the artefacts of past civilizations. Its origins, however, go back far into pre-history, possibly to the legendary Atlantis, or even to an earlier civilization of another 'lost' continent called Mu, whose peoples were also said to be red-skinned.

The Eight-Directions Wheel, like all sacred symbols, had an almost inexhaustible number of meanings and teachings. One was the indication that there were eight times during the year when it was possible to become tuned in readily to the changing rhythms and tides of the Earth's yearly cycle. In Britain and northern Europe in pre-Christian times, for instance, these eight occasions were encapsulated in eight festivals, and the eight-directions circle became the Wheel of the Year.

A pivotal time in the yearly cycle is the *Spring Equinox* on 21 March and this is assigned the *north-east* direction of the Earth Web. It was recognized by the pre-Christian Ostara (Easter) which celebrated the end of winter and the arrival of spring and the coming forth of life again. It was a time of joy because it was the time of sprouting and of everything in Nature coming alive. *The Festival of Awakening.*

The *east* direction heralds the arrival of summer, which was marked by *Beltain* or *Mayday*. The beginning of summer was indicated by the sweet-smelling flowering of the may or hawthorn tree. It was a festival of initiation and the coming into adulthood. It was a celebration of Nature's flowing energy and rising power and so was a time for singing and dancing. *The Festival of Expectation.*

The *south-east* direction marks the longest day, the *Summer Solstice* on 21 June. *Midsummer's Day* was an indication of solar power reaching its peak and the arrival of the long, hot days of summer. *The Festival of Attainment.*

At the *south* we can bask in that summer power which was marked on 1 August by the festival of *Lammas* or *Lughnassad – The Festival of First Fruits, and of Reminder.*

The *Autumn Equinox* (22 September) is the time of balancing and marks the *south-west* point. It was also the time of harvest festivals. *The Festival of Thanksgiving.*

At the *west* we arrive at another pivotal point in the yearly cycle which was considered both as an ending and as a beginning. The ancient Celts regarded it as the time when one year ended and another began and marked it with a festival called *Samhain* (some say it is pronounced 'Sowen') on 31 October. Because it was regarded as the point where winter started, it was looked upon as a doorway between the 'seen' world of matter and the 'unseen' world of the spirit and as a time when powerful natural forces were at work. In popular mythology and superstition it became associated with ghosts and ghouls and it degenerated into Hallowe'en, which has obscured its original importance. *The Festival of Remembrance.*

Moving to the *north-west* we arrive at the *winter solstice* on 22 December. It was marked by a festival that recognized that the seeds that were hidden beneath the surface of the ground and which appeared to be 'dead' and

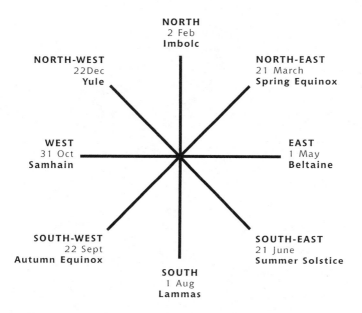

Figure 18. The Wheel of the Year

buried had come alive again and were beginning to stir although their coming to life was not yet apparent. This was the true meaning of *Yule* and the celebrations of a festival which later became known as *Christmas. The Festival of Rebirthing.*

The *north* marked the time for cleansing and purification. The pagan festival of *Imbolc* on 2 February was an occasion for clearing away the dross and dormancy of winter and preparing for the arrival of spring and the freshness of new life. *The Festival of Renewal.*

And so we move round to the *north-east* to complete the round and the arrival of spring and to begin again another turn of the Wheel of the Year.

The eight segments of the Eight-Directions Wheel may be considered to be approximately equivalent to the zodiac signs of Aries, Taurus, Cancer, Leo, Libra, Scorpio, Capricorn and Aquarius. They might have fitted into an Eight-Directions Wheel as shown in Figure 19.

In Sun astrology, the extension to twelve divisions developed through a finer tuning of the system which was made necessary when the range of energies affecting and influencing the human being was taken into account by the introduction of the four Mutable signs.

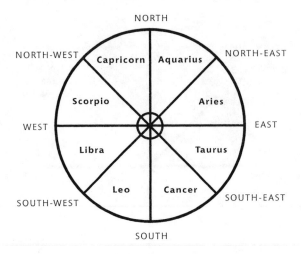

Figure 19. The Ancient Sun Astrology Wheel

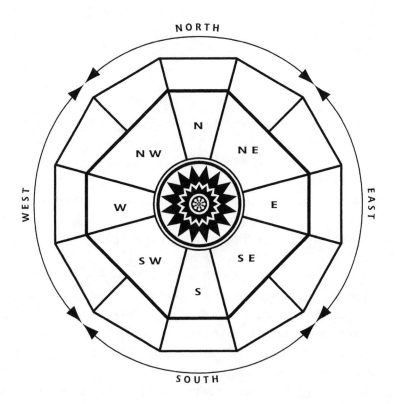

Figure 20. The Twelve Divisions and Eight Directions

In Earth Medicine and present-day Chinese astrology, the remnant of the earlier system is apparent. Each of the Cardinal directions of east, south, west and north occupies one segment, whereas each of the cross-quarters of north-east, north-west, south-east and south-west, covers two segments.

As we construct our Web it is crucial that we grasp the fundamental relationship between the different segments, the four seasons of the natural cycle of the year, and the directional influences because they do affect the way we experience our life on Earth.

The Amerindian might have poetically described the Four Seasons as the coming together of the Sky Father and the Earth Mother. It is all too easy to dismiss such an explanation as simplistically naive, but actually it is quite profound. Perhaps we may better understand it in the context of the yang and yin concept which I began to outline earlier.

The simple symbol used to represent the active, masculine positive yang principle in ancient China was a solid line ▬▬, and the symbol used for the receptive, feminine negative yin principle was a broken line ▬ ▬. The solid line is equivalent to the light, yang, portion of the Tai Chi, and the broken line is equivalent to the dark, yin, portion (see Figure 21).

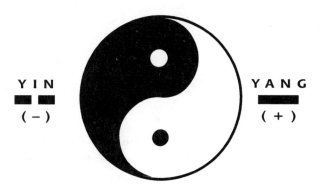

Figure 21.

To help our understanding we can include the (+) positive and the (–) negative signs. We might describe yang as light, so therefore yin is dark. And if yang is hot, then yin is cold.

The union of these two opposites brings into being an 'offspring' which carries the gene of its dominant 'parent' and results in a 'child', a new condition, a separate expression, which can be symbolized in just two lines. So, from the yang ▬▬ (+) Father influence comes 'positive' yang ▬▬

(+ +), which could be described as very bright, or very hot, or *summer*, and 'negative' yang ⚏ (+ –) which could be described as bright becoming dark, hot becoming cold, or *autumn*.

Likewise, from the yin ▬ ▬ (–) Mother influence comes 'negative' yin ⚏ which could be described as very dark, very cold, or *winter*, and 'positive' yin ▬ ▬ (– +), which might be described as dark becoming brighter, cold becoming warm, or *Spring*.

These four symbols in turn produced 'offspring' of eight three-line expressions called *Trigrams*. The trigrams are a further refinement in furthering comprehension of the compositional qualities of the energy or force they represent. They are also a means of access to a vast store-house of ancient wisdom, for they could be compared with the brain-cells of a living entity, or the microchips of a computer. But more about them later. Let us now return to our discussion of the Four Seasons and the Directions with this concept in mind.

We are born into this life during one of the Four Seasons of the year and, according to American Indian cosmology are 'carried' into incarnation, as it were, by the power of whichever of the Four Winds predominates at that time of the year. For instance, in the Northern hemisphere, those born in the spring between 21 March and 20 June are said to be influenced by the warm east winds, people born during the summer 21 June and 21 September by the hot south winds. Autumn people born between 22 September and 21 December come under the influence of the cool west winds, and winter-born people whose birthdays are between 22 December and 20 March with the cold north winds.

Let us understand the meaning behind this. A wind is the movement of air, and can be likened to mind, because mind, like air, cannot be seen. Only its presence can be felt and its power experienced. For instance, the power of Air can be observed by the way the wind sways mighty trees and bends massive trunks and shakes the fruit or seeds from the branches. It has the strength to uproot bushes with a tug and to push huge boulders from their mountain anchorages. Its breath across vast oceans can blow the surface of the sea into foaming, mountainous waves. Anyone who has been outdoors during a severe storm, or at sea in a gale, has experienced the tremendous and awesome power of Air.

According to ancient teachings, the Earth is protected by wind shields which envelope and encompass the planet. These are ascending and descending spirals of movement which are affected by solar and lunar currents. The planet, too, is contained within a cocoon of vibrating electromagnetic energies like the auric egg that surrounds a human being.

The hole in the ozone layer in the Earth's atmosphere which is now the active concern of the governments of many nations is, in fact, a sickness in the Earth's aura which weakens the Earth and is getting worse. As a consequence, there are not merely climatic changes and upsets in the natural seasons and weather patterns, but inhabitants of the Earth are exposed to dangerous ultra-violet rays which the ozone layer screens out. This weakness in the Earth's auric envelope also allows chaotic and disruptive forces to enter, just as would be the case with a human being. These have an adverse and destructive influence at all levels of existence – particularly mental. This, coupled with mankind's wanton destruction of the environment and wildlife, puts the Earth and humanity in grave peril.

The ancient wisdom informs us that the Four Winds are mighty powers that are inherent in the Four Cardinal Directions through which we can be attuned with them. They are mighty powers that affect all living creatures on Earth and especially humans, as well as the atmosphere and the environment.

The Sun and the Moon regulate the ebb and flow of these energies into the Earth's aura. So when we relate to a direction we are aligning our selves with the spin and movement of these mighty forces and their energy expressions.

We cannot see these great powers but we can come to comprehend them through their physical counterparts, and we can experience their influence, for they affect our temperament.

Let us examine how each of the Four Winds affects the direction of our temperament.

As the *east winds* of spring tempt us out into the open after much time spent indoors during the winter months, so the east is associated with *frankness and open-mindedness.*

The *south winds* of summer invite us to spend more time outdoors enjoying the hot summer when everything in the natural world is blossoming and bursting with fragrance. So the south is related to *rapid growth and to blossoming and development.*

The cool *west winds* in the autumn come at a time when growing things have reached their maturity, and harvest time is when we reap the benefit of past labours. So the west is associated with *ingathering and introspection.*

The cold *north winds* of winter purify and cleanse the Earth and force people to spend time indoors and keep warm and to *refresh and renew* themselves.

Each direction is also linked with a time of day – east with *dawn* and the rising Sun of a fresh new day, *south* with *noon* and the Sun at its peak, *west* with dusk and the setting Sun at the end of the day and the time for *reflection and refreshment,* and *north* with midnight and *rest and renewal.*

For those born in the Southern hemisphere the Directions are reversed. Those born between 22 September and 21 December are influenced by the east winds, those born between 21 March and 20 June by the west winds, those born between 21 June and 21 September by the north winds, and those born between 22 September and 21 December by the south winds.

So each of the Four winds and the Four Seasons and the Four Times of Day is related to qualities which have a strong influence on the way we live and even conditions, to some extent, the way we feel and the activities we undertake. And according to American Indian cosmology, the special qualities of the influencing wind or power that predominated and 'carried' us into birth 'rubs off' on us. We carry something of its imprint. It is encoded in us. Absorbed into our brain-cells. Incorporated in the microchips of the bio-computer in our skull.

In the next chapter we are going to examine these qualities and characteristics in detail, together with the signs and totems that represent them and serve as 'switches' that enable us to channel in to them. But first we need to understand something else about the way the American Indians came into a comprehension of abstract concepts and mentative and spiritual principles.

The Indians related everything to what could be observed and understood *from the environment.* Any principle, or natural or cosmic law which affected the life of man – even the mysteries of birth and death and of man's destiny – *could best be understood through observing natural forces at work.*

In order to comprehend an abstraction like a force, a power, an energy, an essence, or an intangible spiritual quality, it is necessary for the human mind to have something to 'grip' onto – a means of containing that elusive intangible in some kind of 'form' so that it might be examined and related to more readily.

The American Indians converted the intangible into a form that could be understood and related to by drawing comparisons with Nature and with the animal, plant and mineral worlds. Wild animals, for instance, shared the environment with them so they were familiar with the individual habits and characteristics of each species, aware of the different temperaments, and saw each animal species as having a personality of its own. They compared the 'hidden' force of Nature and the qualities they had with similar characteristics they observed in certain animals, reptiles, birds or fish. In other words, the Indians 'personified' these intangible forces in much the same way as people in other cultures 'humanized' their gods. The Indians, however, used animals, plants or minerals rather than human representations.

These personifications were called 'totems'. A totem is a special kind of emblem or symbol that expresses the essential *spirit* nature and characteristics not of an individual animal or plant or rock but of the species as a whole and as expressed in the human condition. By being called upon mentally, the totem – whether animal, plant or mineral – becomes a 'spirit helper' to the human being, relating to the human 'spiritually' to specific areas of physical, mental, emotional and spiritual activity. The totems are thus more than psychological symbols. They are active 'helpers' – aids to the human spirit and to an individual's essential nature through the essence of their own essential nature with which the individual has an affinity.

In this way totems make connections with abstract qualities or energies and with other levels of existence. Totems trigger the intuitive senses so that the person who is working with them perceives through the subconscious.

There are other powerful helpers which serve also as representations. The Moon, for instance, can be used as a symbolic representation of the feminine yin, the nurturing Goddess principle. The Moon is *not* the Goddess, but can give us a thrill when we gaze at her. And the Goddess is not a woman, but by responding to her as if she were, we can achieve a connection emotionally with the feminine, nurturing, receptive and tender aspects of the Source. We are thus tuned in, as it were, to receiving an input of energy (information) beamed out from the Source and we can respond to it.

Similarly, the Sun can be used as a symbolic representation of the masculine yang, the God principle behind all Creation. Again, the Sun is *not* the god – and in ancient times, contrary to popular historical theories, the ancients did not *worship* the Sun. The God is not a man, but by responding to it as if it were, we can become aligned to the masculine, creative qualities and we can become attuned to receiving an input of energy (information) on that wavelength.

The totems are different kinds of symbolic representations. They are active, living links that can connect our consciousness to the threads of subtle cosmic forces and natural energies that enter our auric cocoon, the electromagnetic energy field in which we live and move and have our being, and to the delicate but powerful inner forces that ebb and flow between the external 'physical' self and the Real Self at the core of our being.

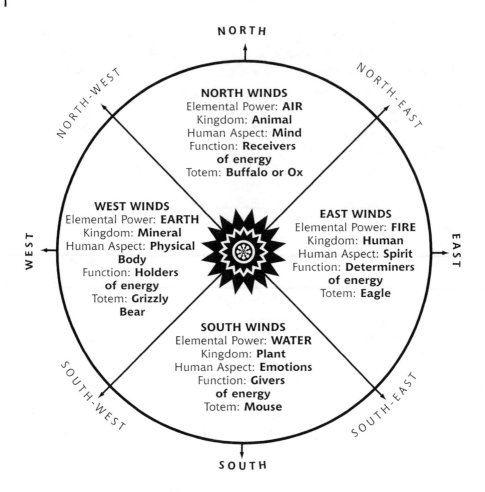

Figure 22. The Powers of the Four Winds

The totems are like transistors in an electronic circuit concerned with directing the flow of energy from one level to another, whether physical (mineral, vegetable or animal) or non-physical (emotional, mental or spiritual). Directional and elemental totems are concerned with cosmic energies from 'above', while other totems are associated with Earth energies which come from 'below'.

Again, contrary to popular belief which was based on ignorance and bigotry, the Amerindian did *not* worship the totems as 'gods' or venerate animals and other creatures as 'gods' or 'demons'. Religious zealots among the early European settlers labelled native practices as 'demonism' and by arousing people's fears of the 'unknown' and inflaming prejudice, encouraged the destruction of what their own ignorance prevented them from understanding.

The totems were but spiritual *tools*. They were honoured and respected for what they represented. The animal representations, for instance, served as a means of comparison. It was not the animal itself though, but its essential quality, its *essence*, which helped in the comparison. The animal itself was a 'helper' because its essential quality which could be recognized, helped the Indian to an understanding of the 'hidden' quality in Nature or in himself with which it was being compared. The creatures chosen to personify or represent the Powers of the Four Winds, for instance, were thus often referred to as 'spirit helpers' or 'spirit keepers'.

There were hundreds of different tribes throughout North America and the creatures chosen as totems were not necessarily identical. The totems given in this book are those which I understand to have been in fairly common use throughout North America as were those indicated to Sun Bear, medicine chief of the Bear Tribe located at Spokane, Washington, through his shamanic vision of the Medicine Wheel.* What is important, however, is that they are ones which people in other lands can readily relate to also.

It is advisable not to be swayed by any argument about which particular animal, bird, plant or mineral is the most appropriate or 'authentic', or which tribe used this and which group of people preferred that. It is what *works* for us personally that matters. Anything else is but a mental or academic exercise. The essential thing is to have 'connections' that 'work' and which trigger an understanding of the concepts that lie behind them. It is the concept that is important and the retrieval of information or manifestation of desired results, not the image itself. *The totem is but a device*, though indeed a spiritual one.

In the next chapter we will examine some of the principal totems and the Directional Powers they represent – the Four Winds – which helped to shape the inner dynamics of our birth.

The Medicine Wheel: Earth Astrology by Sun Bear and Wabun, Prentice Hall Press, New Jersey, USA, 1980.

The Four Winds (1)

T H E   E A S T

THE CREATURE ASSOCIATED WITH THE POWER OF THE *EAST* AND with the East Wind is the eagle. The eagle is a totem for people with birthdays between *21 March and 20 June*. Now let discover how the creature helps us to understand the totem and how the totem helps us to open up our awareness to the Power of the East.

The eagle is a bird that flies higher than any other, so the Indian considered it to be 'closer to the sky'. Of course, such an expression meant something more than its literalism. To the Indian, the sky was synonymous with the realm of spirit and with spiritual things. So the eagle was symbolic of the importance of *principles*. A principle might be defined as a fundamental truth, the essential spirit or intention, or a guide to action.

The eagle is also attributed with remarkable vision. It can see clearly over great distances and identify quite small creatures and objects from a long way off. So the eagle is associated with *far-sightedness* and the ability to look ahead. Since the eagle is also able to look directly into the Sun without being blinded by its intensity, this ability indicates another attribution of the East – *illumination* – illumination which comes to the mind through spiritual vision (remember, the Sun is also a 'living' symbol of divinity or spirituality) or *the ability to see into the essence or spirit of things*.

Eagle feathers were greatly treasured by American Indians because they had helped to carry the bird to great heights where it could be close to the sky (spirit) and from an elevated viewpoint that was detached from the Earth itself and material things, extend its range of awareness. It was able to see more clearly where things on Earth fitted together, and the Indians wanted to acquire this ability for themselves. All too often we are too close to things to understand how they can possibly be part of a meaningful pattern. We go through life like someone trying to make sense of a tapestry or a painting by viewing it from only a few inches away from our nose. Only by taking a position farther away and viewing it from a distance can the picture become clear and the true creativity and intention of the artist be recognized and appreciated. The eagle helped American Indians to acquire more of that ability by tuning in to the 'Spirit' of the East and opening up the mind to that energy.

Each of the Four Winds and the Four Cardinal Directions has a *special relationship* with one of the four principal forms of Earth life which, in Western philosophy and theology, are sometimes referred to as 'kingdoms'. They are: the human, animal, plant and mineral kingdoms. An understanding of this relationship can help us to further the insight we are beginning to develop about ourselves and our Earth.

The special relationship of the East is with the human kingdom. As I have already indicated, the East Winds emphasise *spiritual* considerations and principles, so the 'Spirit' of the East will help us to comprehend more of the *spiritual* nature of the human being rather than the physical, mental or emotional nature.

To the Indian, a human being was far more than just a highly evolved animal – a sort of naked ape with brains! The Indian regarded the human being as a 'divine mortal', or a 'divine physical being'. Indeed, I have had it explained to me that the prefix 'hu' in some tongues meant 'divine', and man, of course, is mortal. So a human being is a divine mortal being – a dual being existing in the realms of both spirit and matter; one spiritual, the other physical; one eternal, the other temporal.

Let us pause here for a moment, for it is important that we bear in mind that the Powers and Forces and Essences we are discussing regarding the Directions, and their qualities and characteristics, are in a moralistic sense, *neutral*. By that I mean that we cannot label them 'good' or 'bad', because they just *are*.

It is the human being who determines the use to which they are put. It is we who determine how the forces and energies shall be directed and used.

Each of us, in our own lives, determines whether we apply our energies in a positive or negative aspect – whether they shall be used constructively or destructively. It is we who determine by the *intent* of their use whether they shall be 'good' or 'bad'. Motive is everything.

The principal function of the East is the *power* of determining – the *power* of making choices. It is the *power* of deciding the way we make use of the energies at our disposal.

With the East concerned with spirit *and* the human being, the Indian concluded that man was in harmony and balance with himself when he *determined* with the *spirit*. That was the way the human being's energy system was structured. Disharmony and imbalance would result if, to use a modern cliché, he 'got his wires crossed' and determined with another part of his being – with the mind, for instance, which is associated with the North, or with feelings, which are associated with the South. This harmonious and synchronous functioning of the entire human being was absolutely vital to well-being. Indeed, health, happiness, abundance and security depended upon it. Finding the right balance between the inner and outer aspects of one's being, between the conscious and subconscious aspects of the mind, and being in tune with the natural and cosmic forces, was to find true contentment and fulfilment, for with that state of equilibrium anything and everything became possible.

Of course, this raises the question: 'What *is* spirit?' There are some very confusing ideas about what constitutes spirit. Some define it as a disembodied soul, or a ghost, others as a force. The Indian's understanding of it was less obscure. Spirit was individuated consciousness expressing itself in differently organized ways.

The Indian saw every entity – including the individual human being – as an individualized spirit expressing its conscious awareness. The human soul was the dwelling-place of the individualized spirit and provided the link between spirit and matter.

The Indian regarded the soul as the storehouse of experience and the seat of the permanent personality that survived all incarnations.

The Indian concluded that as divine mortals, we should determine our actions with the spirit because the spirit was the vehicle of intelligence and had to do with *intentions*. Intentions were related to principles, to ethics and morality, all of which were activities of the spirit. So, even if our 'hearts' are right and we have 'good' intentions, we may still obtain a 'bad' result because we have determined with the mind or with the emotions and feelings and not with the spirit.

Let me give an example. Laws are framed by an activity of the mind and should be designed to establish and safeguard principles (which, as we have seen, are activities of the spirit). It is possible to determine the application of those laws with the mind by keeping strictly to the letter of the law and following its literalism, but be contrary to its spirit and intent. Clever lawyers may find what they call a 'loophole' in the wording of a law that enables them to disregard the intention of the law yet still keep within the letter of the law. The guilty can sometimes 'get away with murder', therefore, on a technicality of law.

Much truth contained in religions whose authority rests on scriptural texts has been sadly perverted and misunderstood in this legalistic way.

We each travel through life at our own pace, making our own choices, and determining in our own way how to exert our own energies in the choreography of our Earth life.

We are, then, each the product of our own determining, creating our own circumstances as we go. We are not the mere robots of Fate.

How do we know when we are determining with the spirit? We determine with the spirit when we follow what the *heart* wants us to do because the true heart is the voice of the spirit.

'We *give* with the heart in order to *determine* with the spirit.' This was the advice given to me by Swiftdeer. That, he explained, was 'the Way with Heart' or 'the Beautiful Way' because it was the way of Love that sought not to exploit or disadvantage others to further self-interest, but rather sought to embrace others in an advantage that could be shared. In that way the Indian considered that one touched oneself and others and even the Earth itself with beauty.

From his understanding of the Four Winds, the Indian concluded that man was composed of all the other 'kingdoms'. His flesh, blood, bones and marrow, and the waters of the body, contained life from the mineral world, life from the plants and their fruit and seed as well as their substance, and life from the flesh of animals. So man was not merely a *part* of the physical world – the physical world, which included minerals, plants and animals, was literally a part of man. Man was a miniature solar system, a microcosm of the universe. Understand man and you understand the Earth and the universe. Understand the Earth and its environment and you understand both man and the universe.

The Real You is the spirit entity that existed before your present Earth life and will continue to exist after your Earth death. The spirit is the inner self that is the eternal you. It is ageless. An elderly person understands the reality of the ageless self. Only the very young think that you feel different as you get older – that somehow the consciousness feels much older at 60 than at 16, that with old age the consciousness gets feebler alongside the body. The truth is that although our ideas and opinions may change with the maturity of the years, we remain the same conscious, individual entity that doesn't feel any different. The body may not be so physically capable, and its limitations may bring frustration, but you are as you have always been – you. Age does not change it, nor does death. Death is merely a change of consciousness.

So what is the purpose of it all? In general terms, the American Indian understood the purpose of life was to expand and magnify the Real Self. The purpose of life was the continuing evolution of the divine spirit within.

The purpose of life, then, is the education of the spirit.

Now let us go back to our examination of the Earth Web. Although people born in the same Earth influence time segment will share similar directional influences and qualities, *they will not be identical.* Though they will share the same emblemic totem – in the case of people born between 21 March and 20 June, for instance, the eagle – I must stress again that it is not just a two-dimensional image printed on the page of a book, or a representation, or indeed the creature itself. The totem is indicative of a mobile, fluctuating cosmos in itself, governed by its own internal dynamics. So whilst we may share similar influences, the effect is determined by the degree of exposure to those influences and also to the level of our internal responses to them.

We have just discussed what spirit is and that the Indian defined it as the essence of the real entity. Your spirit, then, is the essence of the *Real* You.

Now the Indian accepted the reality not only of a life after death, but of a life *before* birth. Nature was his witness to the veracity of that. Before new life sprang forth in the Spring there had to be life before it, and life before that, and so on. Each life in whatever form produces the seeds for its self-perpetuation. Life must go on. That is a cosmic law. Does it not follow that if there is life after death, there must have been life before birth?

The Indian went beyond that, believing that the seeds of the life now being lived were sown in a previous life, and the seeds of the next life were already being prepared by the way the present life was being lived. In other words, there was no real escape from the consequences of our actions. Sooner or later the past does catch up with us!

It follows, then, that we had conscious existence before we were born. Why do we not remember? Because we start each life with a clean 'memory tape'. Using a computer analogy, a clean, new tape is inserted in Drive with each new life. But the 'master' tape is still held in the memory bank of the unconscious of the Real Self. Access to it is normally denied, though there are people who have an ability to recall past-life experiences – who have cracked the past-life recall code.

The directional totem is only one of a number of totems that comprise the personal shield. Each totem is connected with a different part or level of our total being. Each serves as a channel between the outer, everyday conscious existence and the inner reality of our subconscious and unconscious existence. Like a push-button tuner on a radio, it helps us to switch on to a particular wavelength of our being, or like a key on a computer keyboard it enables us to have access to a particular 'menu' of information and energies.

Another of these several totems is our birth totem which is related to the particular time of our birth and provides a finer tuning of the forces and energies that comprise our personality vehicle. For a person born between 21 March and 19 April, for instance, the birth totem is the Falcon; for someone born between 20 April and 20 May it is the Beaver, and for the birth month 22 May – 20 June it is the Deer.

The birth totem is similar to the 'signs' or glyphs used in Sun astrology – for Aries, Taurus and Gemini, for instance – and, indeed, in some ways relates to them. But as I have already indicated, a totem is more than a glyph or a sign on a package of information, it is an activating two-way 'switch' by which we can be directed to our inner levels and through which those inner reaches can filter through to our outer levels to become part of our everyday, physical lives. The birth totem will be dealt with in detail in Part Two of this book.

Each segment of Earth influence time has been allocated a name that describes a feature of Nature's cycle that is evident during that period of the turning of the Wheel of the Year. Briefly, the three segments of the East and their totems are:

The Awakening Time (21 March – 19 April). The principal totem, or birth totem for those born in the Awakening Time is the Falcon which correlates to the Sun sign of Aries.

The Growing Time (20 April – 20 May). The birth totem for the Growing Time is the Beaver, which correlates to the Sun sign of Taurus.

The Flowering Time (21 May – 20 June). The birth totem for those born at this time is the Deer, which correlates to the Sun sign of Gemini.

To summarize: The East is primarily the direction for insight into spiritual principles, so East-born people are likely to be drawn into life-situations in which principles are of prime importance to them and to the direction of their lives. The power of the East expresses itself through the spirit by motivating a desire for new beginnings and new interests, so the response in the individual is an urge to start new projects and to take up new interests (see Figure 23).

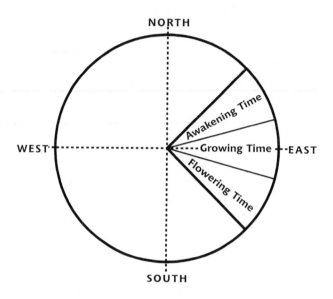

Figure 23.

The Four Winds (2)

S O U T H ,   W E S T   A N D   N O R T H

The South

AN ANIMAL ASSOCIATED WITH THE POWER OF THE *SOUTH* AND WITH the South Winds is the *mouse*. The mouse is a totem for people with birthdays between *21 June and 21 September* in the Northern hemisphere.

A mouse may seem to be a rather unsuitable creature to serve as a totem for a great power. What's more, it is an animal that is not well regarded and may even be feared by some people, and certainly most would regard it as a pest. So why should it be rated as a totem? Bear in mind that to the Indian *every* creature, whether large or small, whether it flew, ran, crawled or swam, had something of value to offer and to teach. There was a reason for its existence. So let us not dismiss the mouse or underrate its likely value as a helper in Earth Medicine. Indeed, little mouse does have much wisdom to impart to us.

The mouse expresses an important characteristic of the 'spirit' of the South because it is a creature that is particularly sensitive to its immediate surroundings through special organs of touch – its whiskers.

Consider how the mouse perceives things. It is aware of its surroundings by its *closeness* to them and by its sensitive *feel* of them. That is a special quality of the South Power and of people influenced by the South Winds – the perception of things by getting close to them. It is a special sort of awareness that comes through *feelings*.

Touch, and closeness, and feelings, are vital qualities of the South, which might be described as the direction of *experience* on the Medicine Wheel. We can't adequately experience anything unless we are somehow touched by it, or unless we allow ourselves to express our feelings and emotions.

The mouse is near to the ground and near-sighted. It sees only the things that are right in front of its nose. People influenced by the South, and especially those born between 21 June and 21 September are like that – seeing mostly only that which is right in front of their noses.

On the other hand, the influence of the 'spirit' of the South can help us all to find our balance because it does stress the importance of not looking so far ahead that one overlooks what lies directly within touch – and perhaps we are all prone to making that mistake.

The mouse is one of the smallest of animals and as such expresses another important principle of the South: never confuse size with true value. After all, our own physical life began from a single cell of an infinitesimal size. A mighty oak tree grows from a tiny acorn. Even the largest enterprises have started from quite small beginnings, and the greatest successes often have their origins in the tiniest incidents.

The South's special relationship is with the *plant kingdom* – the form of life which includes trees and plants, herbs and flowers, and vegetation of all kinds. Trees, especially, are a vital and essential part of the Earth's environment and forests act like lungs to the planet, breathing in carbon monoxide gases that human and animal life expel and exhaling oxygen which human and animal life need to inhale.

Trees and plants provide the animal and human kingdoms with much of their required nourishment. Flowers, herbs and plants have medicinal properties for soothing and healing and restoring the body to a proper balance so that it can function effectively.

We discovered in our study of the East that the principle function there is of determining. In the South the main function is of *giving*, and the plant kingdom contains the great *givers* of the Earth, giving entirely of themselves to provide for other life-forms.

The forms of life that comprise the plant kingdom are thus man's helpers and teachers, too. Essentially, they are endeavouring to teach us the necessity of giving – not of *things* that can be bought and exchanged but rather of *ourselves* which is the only giving of any *real* value. Without the giving of the plant kingdom, we could not survive and physically would wither and die. Without giving we cannot grow, develop and evolve spiritually, but would wither and 'die' spiritually. The Indian knew that. Educated, sophisticated, scientific modern man has moved away from closeness to Nature and has lost touch with that knowledge. The South Direction can help us individually to regain it.

South-influenced people and those born between 21 June and 21 September are likely to have an affinity with plants. They like to have plants around the house, and enjoy gardening or being in gardens. They may feel drawn towards trees and woodlands and find inner harmony by walking in woods and forests.

South people are also likely to feel drawn towards herbal remedies for physical health problems, and to flower remedies in times of stress and when under psychological pressure. Of all people, those most influenced by the South are likely to derive the greatest benefit from these remedies.

In the human world, the South's influence is on the *emotions* and *feelings*. So – applying the principles we have already learned – harmony within ourselves can be attained by *giving* with the *emotions*. All too often we have our 'wires crossed' again. Many of us are afraid to express our emotions because we fear vulnerability. So we hold ourselves back from expressing our true feelings. Love, fondness, appreciation, are more often expressed in the giving of some physical object. There is nothing wrong in that, and I am certainly not advocating that we should dispense with giving gifts, but they are only *tokens*. We need also to give of ourselves but often fail to do just that, so we hold on to our emotions and feelings.

Worse still, when dealing with loved ones, we seek to *hold* on to our emotions and give *with* our minds, when we should *give* with our emotions and hold in our minds.

Love is more than a physical expression, though in our complex consumer society, love – which is a *spiritual* quality and expresses the soul – is stripped of all that to become a mere *physical* expression, so that even the

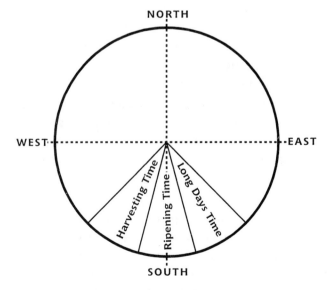

Figure 24.

sexual act is measured or evaluated by mere athletic performance. Love is a *giving* of oneself. Feelings express love. By locking up our emotions and feelings we lock up our hearts and suffer the consequences.

Briefly, the three times of the South are:

The Long Days Time (21 June – 21 July). The totem is the *Woodpecker*, which correlates to the Sun sign of Cancer.

The Ripening Time (22 July – 22 August). The totem is the *Salmon*, which correlates to the Sun sign of Leo.

The Harvesting Time (22 August – 21 September). The totem is the *Brown Bear*, which correlates to the Sun sign of Virgo.

The Power of the South expresses itself through the feelings the individual has of the self. Often the response has been to build myths about oneself and one's feelings.

The Power of the South also expresses itself through feeling the need for events to move forward rapidly. Such traits will be shared by those born between 21 June and 21 September.

The West

An animal associated with the Power of the West and with the West Winds is the *grizzly bear*. The grizzly bear is a totem for people whose birthdays are between *22 September and 21 December* in the Northern hemisphere.

The grizzly is the strongest of all the bears. Self-sufficient, it lives by its own strength, even healing itself of most illnesses and injuries through its knowledge of herbs and its closeness to the Earth.

So the Power of the West is an influence that urges self-sufficiency and the development of the kind of strength that comes from within and which is the most powerful strength of all. West people born between 22 September and 21 December are generally endowed with a degree of inner strength with which to cope with all of life's difficulties, but often need to recognize that it is there for them to drawn upon when needed. They also possess a greater degree of self-sufficiency than most, and are more introspective. They may also feel drawn towards natural healing and complementary medicine.

The grizzly hibernates in winter and makes careful preparation during autumn for the long sleep ahead, eating well and building up its strength, so that when spring comes it will be ready for the time of reawakening and renewal. So the West is the power behind the need for preparation and for gathering in – whether it be the fruits and rewards of past activity, or information and knowledge – before undergoing a period of refreshment or barrenness preceding a new direction or a fresh enterprise.

West people make good gatherers, collectors and storers of things which can be retrieved later and used for further progress.

The grizzly arrives at its decisions slowly and carefully and, in spite of its awesome strength, has a gentle side to its nature. The West is the direction for 'looking within' to examine past actions and to learn from them so that future decisions may be wise ones. It is also concerned with looking within the heart to examine true intentions.

The special relationship of the West is with the *mineral kingdom*; the principal function is of *holding*; and rocks, stones, gems and mineral substances are the great holders and storers of energy.

The mineral kingdom is the most ancient of the four great life-forms on Earth, for rocks and stones were here long before there was vegetation or animals and humans. The Indian believed that when the Earth was in its embryonic state, the primitive rocks developed like the human skeleton to become the Earth's 'bones'. Gemstones were likened to sense organs and quartz crystals to brain-cells.

It was from the ancient knowledge that certain gemstones were related to parts of the *physical body*. For instance, in the ancient wisdom, peridot was related to the eyes and with seeing, onyx to the ears and with hearing, carnelian to the hands and with touch, topaz to the tongue and with taste, jaspar to the nose and with smell. The reason was that these gemstones were connected with the Earth's own sense 'organs' of sight (direction), hearing (the input and sampling of sound vibrations), touch, taste and smell.

Quartz crystal was highly regarded by the Indian, who considered it had special properties as a transformer as well as a storer of energy. The tribal shaman used stick-like pieces of quartz crystal as healing wands. It is not without significance that quartz is an essential substance in the manufacture of computers, calculators, timepieces, and so on.

Modern science has discovered that quartz crystal contains the same chemical composition S_1O_2 as silica, which is a natural mineral within the human body. Silica is concerned with balancing the energy field within the human aura just as strategically placed deposits of quartz around the Earth's surface were believed to balance the Earth's electromagnetic fields. The human body is dependent on essential inorganic minerals and any physical disorders may be due to deficiencies of these energy-storing minerals.

When you hold a piece of quartz crystal in your hand, you are in touch with something that has been in existence long before man first appeared on Earth. And this, of course, is true of all rock. Just reflect on this as you hold a piece of quartz or other natural gemstone and you will come to appreciate why the American Indian had such an affectionate regard for 'Grandfather Rock'.

The emphasis of the West is on apparently 'solid', physical things, so in the human world its influence is on the *physical body*. Our physical body is what *holds* us here as a part of the Earth. We are each the centre of our own universe within the human aura which is similar in a way to a space capsule. In it we can explore and experience the realm of physical matter.

The human physical body is a complex and highly sophisticated piece of equipment – a far greater wonder than any man-made space vehicle. Indeed, it is *the* most wonderful vehicle that has ever been devised!

Just think you grew from a cell smaller than the point of a pin. That cell was like a miniaturized microchip, so tiny that it was invisible to the human eye, yet it contained a program, a genetic code, which contained the image of what you were to become. This program, this image, was eventually objectified into physical form with body, head, legs, arms, facial features, hands, feet and vital organs all of which developed in accordance with cosmic and natural laws. And all within itself!

The genetic code is a system of transmitting information between cells and is embraced within a mathematical structure of binary progression to the 6th power – that is 2, 4, 8, 16, 32 and 64. The genetic code from which you were physically structured produces 64 codons or code 'words'. The Medicine Wheel on which the Earth Web is based is also structured in a similar harmonic way. So is the oriental I Ching which is composed of 64 hexagrams. So is the ancient Circle of Life and Power.

In that genetic code were packed the instructions for building the organic bio-computer that is your brain whose components would be packed together and contained within a protective casing which would also be the seat of normal, everyday consciousness – the skull. The skull itself is an octave of eight bones, like the basic octave of the Medicine Wheel and the Earth Web and of the Circle of ancient 'Mind' Science. That is why it was revered as a symbol by the ancients. Only 'civilized' man turned it into a sinister object. The skull is the container of the brain, which is the bio-computer driven by the mind.

What put that genetic code there to produce such a marvel and such a wonderful physical vehicle for you? *Intelligence* put the program there. It didn't just 'happen'. It was no conceptual 'accident'. There was *intelligence* behind it – and give that intelligence whatever name you wish. Can you still believe that your birth was just an 'accident'?

That first cell of yours was like a microchip – a tiny electronic circuit that had the capacity to memorise and to process and circulate information – a whole, fantastic 'universe' of information and all contained within a simple code. And it did so *instantly*.

Yet for all its awesome wonders, that physical body of yours is but a vehicle of expression. It is not you, only your servant – a means of transporting you about and enabling you to function on the Earth and within the physical realm of existence. Never, after this, *devalue* yourself or your body!

We have seen that the principal function of the East is of determining, and the function of the South is of giving. The function of the West is of *holding*.

Now 'holding' does *not* mean freezing or imprisoning something in order for it to stay as it is. The ancients regarded holding as a reflective pause before change or transformation. 'Holding' is a pause in the transfer of energy – from giving to receiving, or from receiving to giving. It is the 'bit in the middle'. It is an *acceptance* of what has been received whether through one's own efforts or from others, and a consideration of what one can *give* of oneself to keep the 'Wheel' turning.

The West Direction is likened to autumn, which is the season of consolidation when growth stops and when, in the natural scheme of things, humans held onto and stored the fruits of their endeavours and also examined themselves to discover what changes were needed to make progress when the time of renewal came.

This, indeed, is the essence of many life-experiences that West people will find themselves undergoing.

The Power of the West expresses itself as a stabilizing influence. The human response is to gather things around, to get things organized with clear directions or rules and conditions – to have things 'cut and dried'. People born between 22 September and 21 December will share this trait.

Briefly, the three Times of the West are:

The Falling Leaves Time (22 September – 22 October), whose totem is
   the *Crow* and which correlates to the Sun sign of Libra.

The Frost Time (23 October – 22 November), whose totem is the
   Snake and which correlates to the sun sign of Scorpio.

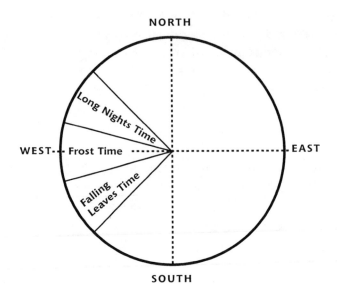

NORTH

Long Nights Time

WEST -- Frost Time

Falling Leaves Time

EAST

SOUTH

Figure 25.

The Long Nights Time (23 November – 21 December), whose totem is the *Owl* and which correlates to the sun sign of Sagittarius.

The North

The creature associated with the Power of the *North* is the *buffalo*. The buffalo is a totem animal for those born between *22 December and 20 March* in the Northern hemisphere. In northern Europe and Britain in ancient times its equivalent would have been the wild, bison-like ox or auroch.

The buffalo was the most important of animals to Plains Indians of old because it supplied everything needed to sustain life. Its meat was food, its hide was material for clothing and for the tipis which were the homes of people. Its bones were made into needles and knives and into cooking and eating utensils. So the buffalo was regarded as an animal that gave of its entirety so that others might have life, and was so likened to the Great Spirit that gives totally of itself to provide the substance for all that exists.

So the North is linked with sustenance. It is also associated with the mind and with knowledge and its power was sometimes described as 'the power of sustenance that knowledge can bring'.

A very rare animal was the white buffalo, which was regarded as a sacred messenger because, according to legend, it was the White Buffalo Woman who gave the sacred pipe to the American Indian people. The sacred pipe is the Indian's most treasured possession.

In Europe, the wild ox was associated with power and tenacity. Its horns were prized as drinking vessels.

The special relationship of the North is with the *animal kingdom* which the Indian classified into four-leggeds, two-leggeds, swimmers, crawlers and winged ones.

We need to appreciate that the Indian did not regard animals as inferior creatures in the way we may do. They were expressions of the Great Spirit, just as man is, and have a spirit also, but they have a different way of *knowing* – a way we might describe as *instinct*. Animals experience the physical environment just as intensely as humans but in a more restricted way because animals are not gifted with free will but motivated by instinct. Their consciousness works differently, being more developed than man's in some areas and less than man's in others.

The Indian observed from animal behaviour how closely animals were in touch with trees and plants and with the elements, and how they moved away from areas of impending danger often long before the danger became apparent. Animals also sensed impending changes in the weather long before a changing weather pattern appeared in the skies. By recognizing these things, Amerindians acquired something of the animal's ability and thereby extended their own field of awareness. The Indian learned much about herbal treatments through observing how animals were guided to certain plants to cure their own wounds or sickness and discovered they were equally effective with humans.

We, too, can learn much from animals. Anyone who has owned a cat or dog, for instance, will have personal experience of how an animal can bring not only comfort and love, but loyalty and understanding. Animals have so much to teach us if only we will cease to exploit them and spend more time in watching and listening.

The principal function of the North is *receiving*, and animals were regarded as the great receivers of energy which they were able to transmit to humans, thus becoming the great *helpers* of mankind. Sadly, though, the animal kingdom has been mercilessly exploited through man's greed and ignorance and the point has now been reached where not only whole species of animals have become or are becoming extinct, but man's very survival is threatened, too, and largely because mankind in general has lost touch with Nature.

The *human aspect* of the North is the *mind*. The mind is not the brain.

The brain is merely a tool of the mind. The brain is physical, material, a bio-computer confined within the protective shell of the skull. The mind, however, is not physical, is not material, but invisible and unconfined. The mind can go anywhere. The brain keeps us alive, but the mind directs our aliveness. The brain emits energy that can be measured. The mind has energy which cannot be measured, only *experienced* as consciousness. The energy of the mind goes where the consciousness goes.

The North is the direction of the mind and the things of the mind – of knowledge and wisdom. Knowledge that is not the kind of useless information displayed by contestants in television quiz games, but the knowledge that can be transformed into wisdom in the Game of Life. And what is wisdom? To the Amerindian, it was *applied* knowledge. It was knowledge applied with love. Whilst knowledge provides answers to the questions: what, when, where, who, and how? – only wisdom explains *why*.

It is not enough to seek knowledge in order to appear knowledgeable and to feed vanity. Nor is it enough to seek knowledge merely as a stimulant for the mind. Knowledge is only of value to the *Inner* Self when it is transformed into wisdom by love, which means by balancing it with the polarity of the South. It is finding this balance and harmony that is part of the purpose of life. We balance and harmonize our own individual inner dynamics by the way we express those energies in the choreography of life which is the way we live.

The Power of the North expresses itself through the mind, and the human response is the way we mentally approach life's challenges and by the beliefs held and the philosophy of life. The mind is a great innovative source, so North people born between 22 December and 20 March are likely to be creative and innovative. Without warm-heartedness, however, they can be aloof, and without compassion they can be calculating and devious. The underlying drive is to encourage them to seek closer rather than superficial contact with others although this may cause them to have to cope with the problems which close relationships generate, but this is part of their learning and growing process.

The North Winds are associated with winter and when the Earth is dormant, so they are seen as the bringers of purification and of refreshment and renewal. Likewise, they were seen as the Power that brings life-experiences that will purify and renew the mind in human affairs. Since the coldness of the winter winds forces us to spend more time indoors, their influence is to bring attention to 'internals' rather than 'externals' and of making effective use of time as a preparation for the period of rapid growth and development which lies just ahead.

In some cultures the North Winds were personified as an Ice Goddess who had the power to turn water into ice and to crush huge rocks into tiny pebbles with the iciness of her breath, but who although appearing outwardly frozen inwardly had a heart of warmth and compassion.

North people have an inner strength and power to change fluid and uncertain situations into solid and more permanent arrangements, but must learn to do so not with cold practicability but with warmth and compassion by allowing their feelings to flow more freely so their spiritual development will not be frozen.

Briefly, the three Times of the North are:

The Renewal Time (22 December – 19 January), whose totem is the *Goose* and which correlates to the Sun sign of Capricorn.

The Cleansing Time (20 January – 18 February), whose totem is the *Otter* and which correlates to the Sun sign of Aquarius.

The Blustery Winds Time (19 February – 20 March), whose totem is the *Wolf* and which correlates to the Sun sign of Pisces.

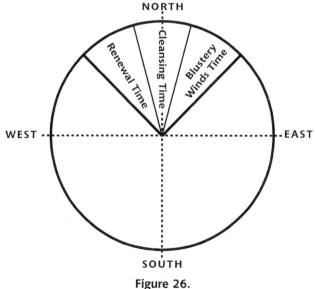

Figure 26.

The Personal Rainbow

EACH OF US IS SURROUNDED BY OUR OWN INDIVIDUAL RAINBOW of colours. But ordinarily, this pulsating band of colours from the energy field in which we are immersed is vibrating at wavelengths that are beyond the comparatively limited range of our normal physical vision. We cannot see these vibrations of colour because they are moving too fast or too slow to come within the range of normal sight.

It is possible with special equipment to photograph a narrow band of radiations around the human body and around animals and plants by a process called Kirlian photography, named after the Russian researchers Sennyon and Valentina Kirlian who made a deep study of the energy fields that surround all living things.

Some highly sensitive people are able to see the auras of other people without the aid of special equipment, but it is usually under certain conditions – after a period of deep meditation perhaps, or shamanic activity, using a method of attunement that has expanded the range of vision. (This has happened to me on occasions, and it is certainly a most wonderful experience to observe for several minutes the shimmering gossamer-like cocoon of a human aura. Others have an ability to sense an aura and, indeed, most people can he shown how to *feel* it.)

But what *is* colour? Colour has been defined as the wavelength of light emanating from or reflected by an object. Colour is light dispersed into a spectrum of rays, each of which has different characteristics and produces a sensation on the retina of the eye which is interpreted as colour.

So the source of colour is light, and colours are different rates of vibrating *light* within an energy system. Light is white – the yang, the primeval Father. Darkness is black – the yin, the 'womb', the primeval Mother – from which all colour comes when penetrated by light.

Colour, like sound, is arranged in a harmonic system, and each colour is divisible into octaves of tints and shades. A tint is any colour with white, and a shade is any colour with black. Each colour, therefore, can have an octave of tints and an octave of shades.

There are three primary colours: magenta (red), yellow and blue. Each of these three primary colours contains white, but only two (red and blue) contain black.

These three primary colours diversify into a spectrum of responses and move in a rainbow pattern from the lowest frequency at the base – which is red – to the highest frequency at the crown – which is violet.

The red end of the spectrum, with its longer wavelengths, is moving towards absorption and the black (yin) polarity, whilst violet has a shorter wavelength and is moving towards the white (yang) polarity – separation and individuality. Magenta is where the octaves change.

So the sequence is from magenta through red, orange, yellow, green, blue and indigo to violet.

Colour is what our senses perceive to exist between light and dark; between what can be seen and what is invisible. There are colours our senses do not see between what is manifest and what is unmanifest. Colour is where we are touched by that part of the Creation that has either become visible and manifest or is about to be absorbed. In other words, colour is where change is taking place. And change is the only *constant* factor in the universe.

When colour strikes the surface of an object or being, some of its rays are absorbed into that object or energy-system. So colour not only affects the appearance of things but the energy of the energy-systems it touches. Colour also has a psychological effect on us as individuals.

At the positive end of the polarity spectrum, white (yang) is reflective and stimulating and represents the active forces of life – force and spirit, whereas at the receptive end of the polarity, black (yin) is the passive and absorptive energy of life – form and body. Movement is always from yang to yin (+ to –).

The wavelengths towards the receptive (yin) polarity are longer, with a slower vibration and a heavier 'feel' than those at the positive (yang) end. So red, for instance, is moving more in tune with the physical than say, violet, at the positive end which is moving more in tune with the spiritual.

Colour and sound are aspects of the same thing – the movement or vibration of energy. So sound might be described as colour we can *hear*, whilst colour might be described as sound we can *see*. The matter is, of course, very subjective because, as humans, we have finite visual and audible ranges.

The vibrations of sound are not near those of the visible light band, although the difference between colour and sound is a difference only in the number of vibrations a second. Silver Bear explained it to me in these words:

'In the beginning was the Sound, but the Sound was the sound of the Great Spirit who caused matter to form and to take shape. The sound contained the thought, and thought is silent sound.'

Since colours are energies and we are each of us an energy system, when we are with other people the frequencies (colours) emanating from our own aura are brought into close contact with those emanating from the auras of other people. We find ourselves attracted to some people and not so attracted to others, not because of what may have been said but merely by a 'feeling' we get about them. What has happened is that there is harmony or discord between the colours or vibrations, of the essential qualities of the energy-systems.

Each of the colours of the spectrum I have described is related to a power centre of the Energic Body within the human auric cocoon because that power centre primarily responds to that colour. The electric-like Energic Body is a non-physical subtle body which interpenetrates and extends beyond the physical body, almost like a sheath. These power centres might be described as 'organs' of the Energic Body, and are usually referred to as 'chakras' in metaphysical circles. Chakra is a Sanskrit word which means 'wheel' or 'vortex', and this is a good description because the power centres are wheel-like vortices of whirling energy/light.

My mentors have described them to me as 'luminous power wheels'. The principal ones are approximately in line with the spinal column and are situated at focal points where the strands of light energy, of which the human aura is composed, cross and recross many times.

These power wheels are not part of the physical body, but exist at a non-physical level which some might describe as 'etheric'. Some clairvoyant people claim to be able to see them. Other sensitive people are able to discern them in some other way.

Part of the purpose of these chakras is to take in subtle vital energies – cosmic, Earth and elemental forces – and transform and distribute them to the organs and key centres of the human physical body through the cerebrospinal and parasympathetic nervous systems and the endocrine glands. The endocrine glands are groups of special cells that secrete hormones to the bloodstream. Hormones might be described as chemical 'messengers' that control many of the functions of other cells and tissues.

Each chakra has a particular function. In general terms, those located below the diaphragm are concerned with the mundane activities of physical existence – with our physical survival – and those above the diaphragm with the creative and expressive activities.

Like our physical organs, the chakras can be damaged or impaired. Shock, emotional upsets, fear, stress and anxiety, for instance, can affect their activity and harmonious functioning, and thus the flow of vital forces coming into the energy-system causing a subsequent malfunctioning of the physical body.

Indeed, there is a form of bio-magnetic therapy which can measure the response of the chakras and bring them into harmony and balance where there is a malfunctioning. Some American Indian shamans were able to manipulate the energies of the chakras in a similar way through the use of crystals and gemstones.

The vital force referred to in Hatha Yoga as *prana*, and which some American Indians called *Mana*, is an electric-like 'substance' which is drawn in with the breath or may be extracted from the fresh food and drink we consume. It – or lack of it – affects not only the physical body, but the emotional, mental and spiritual bodies also.

The chart overleaf and Figure 27 provide information on the main chakras, their primary colour responses, and their functional significance.

The number of major chakras listed here differs from that found in books on traditional metaphysical systems. Traditional systems list only seven chakras and this is because they are trapped in history since they were originally related astrologically to only seven planets known to the Chaldean/Hebrew originators (using Mercury, Venus, Mars, Jupiter, Saturn, the Sun – though it is really a star – and the Moon, which is really a satellite). The discovery of Uranus, Neptune and Pluto indicates that this 'traditional' system was incomplete, though 'true' at the time it was formulated. Each chakra or energy wheel vibrates in tune with a planet. Our culture has now developed further from theirs, and we are open to a wider range of energies we can use but which were not available to them. The *ten* chakras listed here are in accordance with an even more ancient wisdom – Egyptian, Atlantean and Amerindian – which, paradoxically, happens to be the most up-to-date for it recognized the existence of these energies.

The three chakras that are additional to the seven 'traditional' ones are the Root chakra, which is situated beneath the feet and whose primary function is *nurturing*, the Feet chakra, which is situated between the ankles and whose main function is *movement* and balance, and the Base-of-the-brain chakra, whose function is *power* and activity.

Consider how the human condition is affected by exposure to these energies. The people of modern, industrial nations, for instance, are more *caring*, compassionate and considerate in their attitudes (the Root chakra power) that was the populace of the ancient Middle Eastern cultures under

Chaldean influence. Today, there is rapid *movement* and transportation from place to place, from country to country, and from continent to continent. Rapid movement has become almost a necessity of life (the Feet chakra influence). Consider the *power* that is now available to the ordinary person – the power that household gadgetry puts within the hands of the average housewife, the power that mechanical and electronic equipment makes available to the average man. Consider the awesome power of communication that television, radio and computer technology places at our fingertips. Each and every one of the these powers and activities we take for granted today, yet in times past the people would have regarded them as beyond the reach of mere mortals. Accessibility to such powers is related to Base-of-the-Brain chakra activity.

Shamans told me that these three chakras once functioned in the human condition in Atlantis and Mu – ancient civilizations of pre-history – but became dormant after the Earth's orbit of the Sun was changed and those civilizations disappeared as a result of the catastrophic effects on the Earth's

TABLE OF CHAKRAS AND COLOURS

Chakra Name	Location	Primary Colour Response	Frequency Multiple	Factors of Frequency Multiples	Functional significance
1 Root	Beneath the feet	Magenta (Red)	1	1 x 1	Nurturing.
2 Feet	Between the ankles	Dark Red	2	1 x 2	Balance and movement.
3 Base	Base of spine	Mid Red	4	2 x 2	Foundation. Elimination.
4 Sacral	Lower intestine and sexual organ area	Orange	6	2 x 3	Motivation and reproduction. Desire.
5 Solar	Solar plexus	Yellow	10	2 x 5	Growth and balance. Will.
6 Heart	Heart	Green	12	2 x 2 x 3	Emotional love, compassion. Fear.
7 Throat	Throat	Light Blue	16	2 x 2 x 2 x 2	Communication.
8 Base of Brain	Base of brain	Mid Blue	36	2 x 2 x 3 x 3	Action.
9 Brow	Forehead	Indigo	96	2 x 2 x 2 x 2 x 2 x 3	Mind-power. Thought. Vision.
10 Crown	Top of head	Violet	972	2 x 2 x 3 x 3 x 3 x 3 x 3	Wisdom and Intuition.

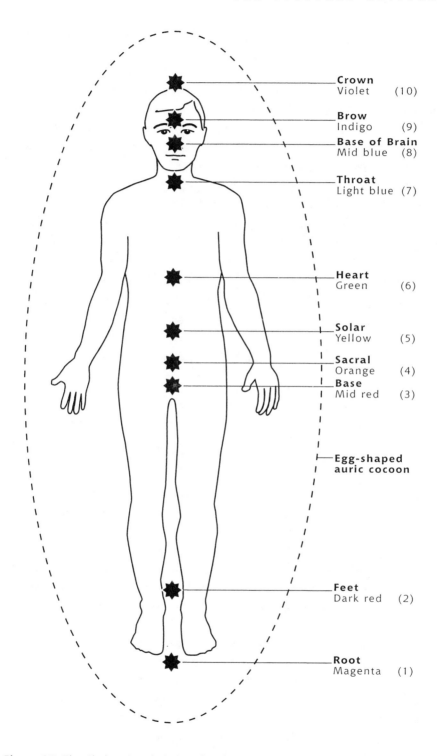

Figure 27. The Chakras in relation to the physical body

surface leaving comparatively few survivors. Knowledge of them and of their eventual reawakening was known, however, to shamans who had access to the ancient wisdom.

The colour of each directional power on the Medicine Wheel – yellow for East, red for South, black for the West, and white for North – is an expression of how its inherent qualities are likely to affect us. Put another way, the colour of a directional power – which, remember, is itself an energy system – is the vibratory rate of the *essence* or spirit of that power.

The individual human spirit absorbs something of the Ray quality of the directional influence and to an extent this will be absorbed and reflected in the aura and in the personality. We absorb such directional ray qualities not only by being born under their influence but through deliberately and consciously seeking them because we need greater exposure to their energies in order to bring our own energy-system into better balance and harmony.

The colours of the Directions of the Four Winds, or Powers, taken in an especially symbolic order are:

NORTH	(Mind)	White	The colour of Intensity. Decisiveness. Penetration.
WEST	(Body)	Black	The colour of solidity. Earthiness. Endurance.
EAST	(Spirit)	Yellow	The colour of Optimism. Stimulation. Exuberance.
SOUTH	(Feelings)	Red	The colour of Energy. Strength. Passion. Courage.

This indicates a semi-gyrating movement which applies to everything and in this case is North to West, and East to South. Movement from North to West is counter-clockwise and from East to South is clockwise. We therefore have two opposing movements which are in a state of dynamic balance at any moment in time (see Figure 28).

When we plot this movement on a chart we are presented with a symbol – the symbol of Wakan-Tanka, the Great Everything. It indicates that from the mind/will of the Great Spirit in the North, energy moves to the West into physical matter, then to the East to appear as a spirit and to be given illumination, and to the South to live life as a Child of Nature, returning energies to the Soul and then back to the Source. This is central to the teaching of the Medicine Wheel.

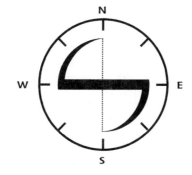

Figure 28.

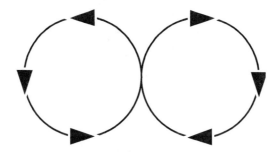

Figure 29. The Wakan-Tanka symbol of perpetual motion indicated by a figure-of-eight movement

The North corresponds to mind, which thinks in forms, and the West corresponds to body, which is concrete form. The East corresponds to spirit, which is a force, and the South corresponds to the Soul and the feeling of forms. So here we have the dynamic balance between force and form in the cosmos. This, therefore, is the symbol of Wakan-Tanka which is everything manifested from the Unmanifest.

The letter 'S' is symbolic of Wakan-Tanka. The figure-of-eight on its side indicates the unending continuity of Life.

The Wakan-Tanka symbol is very similar to the S-Rune of the ancient Northern peoples of Britain, Europe and Scandinavia. The S-Rune ⚡ expresses the life-giving force of the Sun and the forces of light and order. It is also the rune of higher being – the inner spiritual guiding force.

It is not without significance that the four cardinal colours of the Medicine Wheel and the Earth Web are the colours of the four primary races of mankind – the *White*-skinned (North), the *Black*-skinned (West), the *Yellow*-skinned (East) and the *Red*-skinned (South). The colour of one's skin is related to the race one was born into and through which one has physical

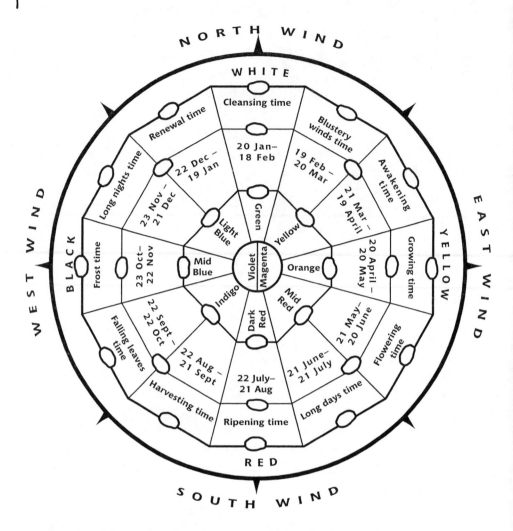

Figure 30. Colours are indicated at the centre of the Earth Web.

ancestry. It 'colours' the perspective one has of life. However, a highly evolved soul can reincarnate into any race it chooses.

No race is superior or inferior to another. They each express a fundamental quality of the Whole and are essential to one another. Each is working at a different aspect of spiritual evolution and each is expressing different ideas through the diverse cultures.

We can now develop our Earth Web a stage further.

The Elemental Powers

W E HAVE NOW CONSTRUCTED OUR TWELVE-SPOKED MEDICINE
Wheel and indicated its Quarters and Cross-quarters. We have also
identified the totems which influence the twelve Time segments and how
the Moon affects each period of approximately thirty days. And we have also
plotted the wind or directional power that influences each of the times and
discovered the colour and 'feel' of each power. So, depending on our date of
birth, we can each locate our own 'starting' place on the Earth Web and in so
doing discover some broad, general traits about ourselves.

Now we are going to examine another factor which has an effect on the
alchemy of our personality – the Elemental Powers and primary 'substances'
of which we are composed and which affect us physically, emotionally, psychologically and spiritually. But in endeavouring to comprehend this concept
of the elemental forces let us again attempt to understand the American
Indian mind.

The 'primitive' Indian had a child-like (though not child-ish) innocence
compared with an 'advanced' and sophisticated modern person who has
been nurtured in a scientific and technological society. Yet the Indian seemed
to have a more profound understanding of the way Nature worked.

The American Indian 'wise men' regarded matter as invisible energy
condensed and 'solidified' into visibility through elemental substances and
directed by intelligence through Elemental Powers. The invisible was thus
made manifest and maintained in being by a directing intelligence within
the Whole. Just as we understand that individual cells and organs of the
human body are maintained by intelligence within them, and the vital
functions of the body are controlled by the subconscious or unconscious
mind of which there is no conscious awareness, so the Indian saw the whole
of Nature operating similarly. He regarded it as the Great Spirit made
manifest. That is why he had such respect and affection for the environment
around him.

Physical science may tell us that there are over a hundred chemical elements from which matter is composed – like oxygen, nitrogen, hydrogen, carbon, and so on. The Indian understood things rather more simplistically, and expressed that understanding more poetically. The Indian might claim that there are four elements in all things and these four – Air, Fire, Water and Earth – are derived from a fifth, the 'Breath of the Invisible' out of which these four come. This is similar to the five-element basis of Chinese medicine and philosophy.

This 'Breath of the Invisible' has a similarity with what some occultists have called Ether or Aether. In esoteric circles it is sometimes referred to as 'the Void'. The name is comparatively unimportant. Its meaning is a quintessence out of which everything comes.

The 'Breath of the Invisible' is also a poetic way of describing the activation of the Life-Force which gives all things their 'aliveness' and conscious awareness. 'Religious' people sometimes refer to this presence under the general label of 'God'. It is eternal because It has been present in the eternity of the ever-present Now that has existed in what has gone before and will exist in what is yet to come. It is infinite because It exists in all things and in all places and is without beginning or ending. It is all-knowing because through Its existence in all things It is the Source from which all things originate.

The Breath of the Invisible, Aether, the Void, is placed at the *centre* of the Medicine Wheel because it is the source of the Four Elements. It occupied the symbolic 'dot' in the centre of the circle, but it is also present in the entire circle because it is in everything. It is the space of the universe as well as the space within the atom. It is That through which come physical manifestations.

The Four Elements are inherent in all manifestation. But they are *not* the physical elements of *real* air, *real* fire, *real* water and *real* earth, but rather the four states or *conditions* of matter. Air refers to *all* gases, Fire to all radiant and electrical phenomena, Water to all fluids, and Earth to all solids. They are the principles behind the physical manifestation – the invisible 'substance' which is in the process of becoming material substance. Physical air, fire, water and earth have the characteristics and nature of the elemental essence, and it is these qualities which we are endeavouring to recognize and understand so that we can apply them.

Air might be described as the principle of *movement*. It cannot be seen, although its presence can be felt and observed by its effect on what it touches. We know not where it comes 'from' or where it goes 'to'. We can track only its movement.

Air is associated with the *North* on the Medicine Wheel because the strongest winds were observed as coming from the north.

Fire might be described as the principle of *expansion* and *transmutation*. Fire is associated with the Sun, that great ball of fire from which the entire solar system derives its light-energy. Since the Sun rises in the east, Elemental Fire is assigned to the *East* on the Medicine Wheel.

Fire energy is expansive.

Water might be described as the principle of *fluidity*. Water flows, and takes the shape of whatever contains it, and finds its own level. Since the movement round the Medicine Wheel is in a clockwise direction, elemental Water is assigned to the *South*.

Earth might be described as the principle of *inertia* and *stability*. Earth is the taking of form, the appearance of solidity. Earth is assigned to the *West* on the Medicine Wheel.

If you are familiar with Sun astrology and Western mystical systems you will have noticed that the Elements are placed in different directions on the Earth Wheel or Web. In Western systems Air is placed in the east, Fire in the south, Water in the west, and Earth in the north. The emphasis is on manipulation. Whereas Earth Medicine places Air in the north, Fire in the east, Water in the south, and Earth in the west. The emphasis in on harmonization.

The Elements are not, of course, confined to a particular direction. Each is present in all directions. The direction indicates influence, not substance.

The placings of the Elements in relation to each other are the same in both systems. Both systems work. The difference is that the Wheel has been moved a quarter turn (see Figure 31). The result is a change of emphasis,

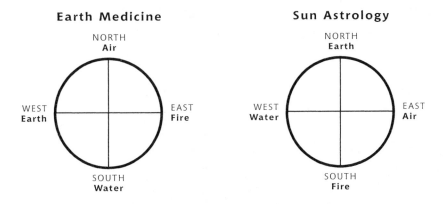

Figure 31. Differences in the 'placings' of the Elements

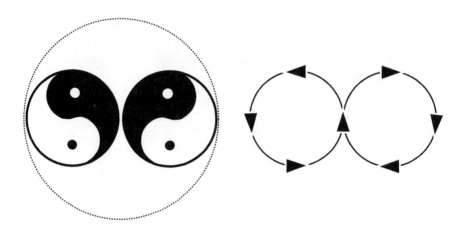

Figure 32. The Infinity Movement and its relationship with the Tai Chi

from subjection and coercion to one of participation and co-operation, and its function is to harmonize the individual with all levels of being.

Earth Medicine is derived from the Medicine Wheel which was known among the ancients as the Creation Wheel – the Key Driver Wheel that drives the 'wheels within wheels' within the spirals of Creation. Within the Creation Wheel was described what was known as the Infinity Movement which I referred to in the previous chapter.

The Infinity Movement (see Figure 32) is a state of perpetual motion and can be represented as a double circle like a figure 8. It describes the interplay of the yang and yin polarities within the unity of the Circle of Power. It is a motion in which the two circles appear to be revolving in opposite directions, one clockwise and the other anticlockwise.

In human terms the Infinity Movement when related to the Medicine Wheel describes the way we each experience Earth life and how we are processing our experiences. In practice most of us become 'stuck' in our perceptions and therefore our understanding is limited and curtailed. We go through a repetition of the same old problems and experiences though wrapped up in different sets of circumstances because that is the way we are subconsciously 'driving' the infinity movement of our own inner dynamics.

Earth Medicine can help us to extend and raise our perspective and to consciously create an infinity movement that will put us in balance and harmony and result in a more fulfilling life.

This does not mean that one system is 'right' and the other 'wrong' or that one is to be preferred as 'better', merely that there is a change of *per-*

spective. One requires the application of complex mathematical calculations and some knowledge of astronomy and in ancient times was the reserve of the learned and of the priesthood. The other requires the observation of the cycles of Nature and attunement with Nature's forces and in ancient times was the province of all.

The essence of Sun astrology is 'As Above, So Below'; the essence of Earth Medicine is 'As Within, So Without'. Sun astrology is a way of looking outwards for explanations – to the stars and the planets; Earth Medicine is a way of looking inwards – to the spiritual Sun and the spiritual Moon within us all.

Sun astrology is concerned with changes that are coming into our sphere of influence – future events; Earth Medicine is concerned with making changes in ourselves in the present so that we can have greater control over our own future. Sun astrology is a looking outside for an explanation of the inside; Earth Medicine is a looking inside for an explanation of the outside.

Let us now consider different ways these elemental powers function and affect the human condition. The elements can be related to the Four Planes of Reality (see Figure 33).

Earth is related to the physical, *Material Plane* of ordinary, everyday reality – the world of matter which is perceived through the five physical senses of sight, hearing, touch, taste and smell.

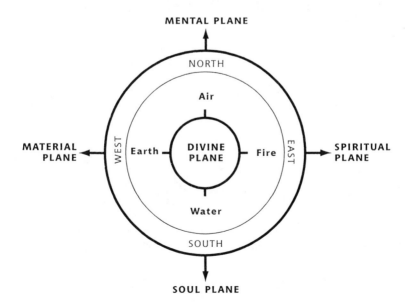

Figure 33. The Wheel of the Planes

Water is related to the *Soul Plane* – the plane of desire – whose reality is perceived through the feelings.

Air is related to the *Mental Plane* – the realm of thought – whose reality is perceived through the mind.

Fire is related to the *Spiritual Plane*, which is perceived through the heart. The Spiritual Plane is experienced through the love that is a giving of oneself. Only through giving itself can the isolated, individual self experience the being of another, and by so doing experience the very essence of life itself.

This concept of the Four Elements enables us to see 'into' things and to recognize the reality that is hidden to the physical senses but which permeates and animates the Realm of Form. Figure 34 shows the Realm of Form applied to the Medicine Wheel.

The concept of the Four Elements can help our understanding of love itself, for it helps us to recognize that there are four types of love that arise out of Divine Love:

Earth relates to physical attraction – physical love.

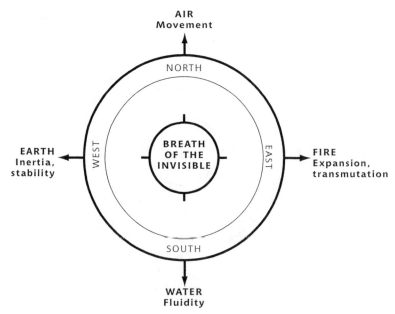

Figure 34. The Realm of Form

Water relates to the urge to merge – sexual love.

Air relates to the brotherly love of friendship – platonic love.

Fire relates to the selfless, non-possessive love that is eternal because it is True Love – spiritual love.

The Four Elements also help us to understand the Constitution of the human being (see Figure 36).

Earth is related to the *physical body* and is associated with the *sensations*.

Water is related to the soul and is associated with *feelings* and *emotions*.

Air is related to the *mind* and is associated with *thinking* – with thoughts and ideas.

Fire is related to the *spirit* and is associated with *intuition* and *inspiration*.

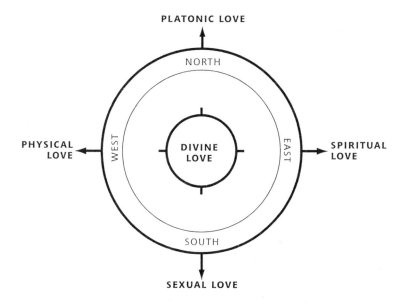

Figure 35. The Wheel of Love

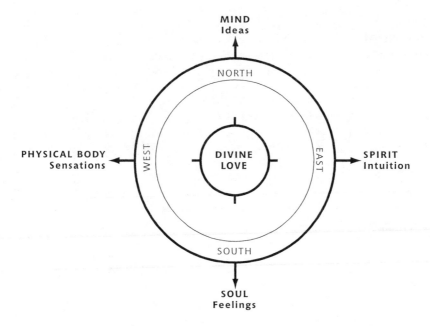

Figure 36. The Wheel of the Constitution of the Human Being

The concept of the Four Elements also helps us to a better understanding of people when we recognize what is predominating.

In other words an element has an essential spiritual nature which can be expressed through all the kingdoms – mineral, plant, animal and human. Earth Medicine shows that North people (those born between 22 December and 20 March) will have, or will be seeking to express, the basic spiritual nature of Air; East people (those born between 21 March and 20 June) will have, or will be seeking to express, the basic spiritual nature of Fire; South people (21 June – 22 September) of Water, and West people (23 September – 21 December) of Earth.

The predominance of an element does not necessarily mean that the nature of that element will be expressed through that individual, only that it is *seeking* expression. Let me give examples:

Air is the great transforming element that is in constant motion. So Air-orientated people may find themselves darting hither and thither, busying themselves in all sorts of activities, or, perhaps, only finding satisfaction when there are plenty of things to do. They need activity or they become bored.

Fire people will have a fiery enthusiasm for almost anything that captures their interest at a particular time, and may find a need to curb a tendency to be so all-consuming that they become possessive.

Water people are likely to be adaptable and easy-going, and may find the necessity of fitting in with their surroundings and with others essential to their feeling at ease.

Earth people may find that stability and the need for security is an essential part of their nature.

The psychological properties of the Four Elements express themselves in the human personality in some of the following ways:

Air stimulates. Air is clear and uncluttered. Air provides impetus. Air is the realm of thought and the intellect, and expresses itself particularly in:

- Mental and verbal communication.
- Ideas.
- Social popularity.

The polarity of Air is yang (+) because it is active and expansive.

Fire energizes. Fire ignites and consumes. Fire is the element of transmutation – it brings about dramatic changes. Fire is the realm of spirituality, of sexuality and passion. It expresses itself particularly in:

- Creativity.
- Enthusiasm and drive.
- Extroverted behaviour.
- Versatility.

The polarity of Fire is yang (+) because it is penetrating.

Water dispenses. Water is fluid and constantly changing. It is the element of absorption and germination. Water is the realm of love and the emotions. Water expresses itself particularly in:

- Imagination.

- Sympathy and understanding.

- Sensitivity.

- Introverted behaviour.

The polarity of Water is yin (–) because it is receptive.

Earth contains. Earth is stability. Earth is the foundation of the Elements and the one we are the most comfortable with because it is stable and solid and dependable. Earth is the realm of abundance and prosperity. Earth expresses itself particularly in:

- Practicalities.

- Patience and persistence.

- Sensuality.

- Conservatism.

- Cautiousness.

The polarity of Earth is yin (–) because it is fertile, nurturing and fruitful.

The elemental forces seek to express themselves in a three-way cycle of activity:

1. The Way of Creating and Initiating.

2. The Way of Preserving or Consolidating.

3. The Way of Transition or Changing.

So the *first* stage of the cycle of activity is *initiatory*. It is getting things going by the application of energy (*Fire*).

The *second* stage is to ensure that what has been started is going to hold and be made more permanent, so what has been started must be *consolidated*. The stability of *Earth* is applied.

The action of Fire on solid Earth produces gas (Air) which, through condensation, becomes *Water*. So the mingling of these two previous stages produces *change*. The *third* stage, then, is Change, or the transition from one condition to another. Water, therefore, follows Air in this cyclic pattern.

The sequence of the Elements in this cyclic pattern within the Wheel is then: Fire, Earth, Air and Water, and the sequence of the three ways of expression is: Creating, Consolidating and Changing. Each element is therefore seeking expression in each of three ways through a sequential pattern that synchronizes with the twelve segments or times of the Earth Medicine Wheel and which themselves are the twelve expressions of personality.

Fire seeks expression through *ideas* – by initiating new ideas, consolidating accepts ideas, and by making changes to ideas to meet fresh circumstances.

Air seeks expression through *communication* – by taking the initiative in communication, by putting into form what has already been communicated and by changing the methods of communication.

Water seeks expression through *ideals* – through formulating and establishing them or through modifying them to suit the changing times.

Earth seeks expression through *work* in its three ways of activity – through initiating work, through completing work, or by changing the way work is done.

People whose birthdays occur in any of the three months in which a particular element predominates have an affinity with each other. The Indian recognized this elemental affinity as an *elemental clan*. A clan is an association of people related by ancestry, and those belonging to an elemental clan are related not by blood but by 'genetic' similarities of the elemental influences whose characteristics they share and which are part of their physical being and determine, to a degree, something of their physiological and psychological make-up which has a bearing on the way life is perceived and expressed.

So, by following the cyclic pattern within the Earth Medicine Web we can identify the clans as follows:

CLAN OF FIRE:

Falcons (21 March – 19 April)
Salmon (22 July – 21 August)
Owls (23 November – 21 December)

CLAN OF AIR:

Deer (21 May – 20 June)
Crows (22 September – 22 October)
Otters (20 January – 18 February)

CLAN OF WATER:

Woodpeckers (21 June – 21 July)
Snakes (23 October – 22 November)
Wolves (19 February – 20 March)

CLAN OF EARTH:

Beavers (20 April – 20 May)
Brown Bears (22 August – 21 September)
Geese (22 December – 19 January)

Totems used in Earth Medicine to represent these elemental clans:

The *Hawk* represents the Clan of Fire.
The *Butterfly* is the totem for the Clan of Air.
The *Frog* represents the Clan of Water, and
The *Turtle* represents the Clan of Earth.

From now on, in dealing with the relationships to the elemental forces operating in their cyclical patterns, I shall refer to them as:

The *Hawk Clan* (Fire).
The *Butterfly Clan* (Air).
The *Frog Clan* (Water).
The *Turtle Clan* (Earth).

Let us now take a more detailed look at the totems and their clans.

The Hawk Clan (Fire)

The hawk is a powerful bird which, like the eagle, can fly to great heights and thus be 'near the Sun'. The Indians also associated the bird with thunder and lightning. So the hawk characterizes the *radiant* energy of Fire, the *sudden illumination* of the flash of light, and the *power* that is inherent in the *transmuting* energy of Fire.

Hawk Clan people often have flashes of inspiration to spark new ideas and projects and a burning enthusiasm that is necessary to activate them. They are usually clear-sighted and energetic people.

Hawk people can gather much strength from the warmth of the Sun and invigoration from being outdoors after a storm when the air has been cleaned and purified.

The Butterfly Clan (Air)

The butterfly was possibly chosen as the totem for elemental Air not merely because it is a creature that is constantly *moving*, always *active*, always shifting its position from one place to another, but because of its great *transforming* powers. For what was an unattractive crawling insect, slow-moving and vulnerable, turns into a most beautiful and delicate flying creature that weaves rainbow patterns in the air.

Butterfly Clan people are always active – either physically, mentally or emotionally – with fresh ideas and often unexpected ways of doing things. They are manipulative and like to transform things.

Butterfly Clan people have an affinity with air, so they will be invigorated and stimulated by being out in big open spaces and away from any kind of confinement whenever possible.

The Frog Clan (Water)

The frog was chosen as a totem for the Water Clan because it is a creature that undergoes dramatic changes in its development from a tiny, swimming tadpole with only a tail to a four-legged creature which is able to adapt itself to the quite different environment of land.

The frog characterizes elemental Water because of its *adapatability* and *flexibility* in undergoing change and its ability to fit in with its surroundings. But the frog lives mostly in water which is likened to feelings and emotions and Frog Clan people, too, are affected more by feelings and because of their sensitivity have an empathy towards others.

Frog Clan people have deep emotions, and like flexibility and malleable arrangements rather than rigid situations. They like to be able to determine how the tide of events is flowing and to move with it.

Frog Clan people have an affinity with water and can find calmness and a soothing effect from being near water – the sea, a lake, river, stream or even a pond in the garden. So they should seek to be near water as frequently as possible.

The Turtle Clan (Earth)

The Turtle is a creature of water as well as of the land, and as it swims in the water its shell looks like the land rising up out of the sea. The Turtle is characteristic of elemental Earth because of its *solidity* – its hard protective shell providing *warmth, comfort* and *security*. The Turtle may appear to be slow-moving but its *persistence* and *tenacity* get it to where it wants to go.

Turtle Clan people are usually methodical, practical and down-to-earth. They like to have a sureness about things and the security of something solid behind them. They have determination, but make progress a step at a time.

Earth Clan people have an affinity with the Earth itself and with plants and growing things. They can find revitalization by visiting a park or woodland or some natural place with things of the Earth around them.

I must make it clear that none of us are affected by only one element. The element of our elemental clan and of the directional power will be the one or ones with which we have the greatest affinity. But as everything in physical existence is composed of a combination of elements operating in different proportions, so it is with us psychologically, emotionally and mentally. Once the basic combination of ourselves is known, we have a key to understanding more about our own inner dynamics and how to harmonize with them and keep them in balance. And, of course, such knowledge can help us to understand and relate more easily to others.

Figure 37 places the Elements on the Earth Web.

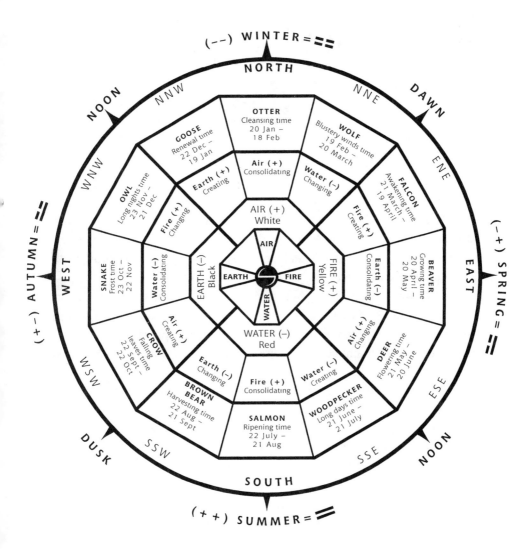

Figure 37. The placing of the Elements on the Earth Web

The Wheel and the Web

IDESCRIBED EARLIER HOW THE YANG AND YIN FORCES INDICATED the primordial duality in Nature and are reflected in the Four Seasons and the Four Directions. This spiritual 'sexuality' is expressed also through the elemental powers to permeate everything that is manifested.

Let us now develop the yang/yin concept further, from the duality principle of the Four Symbols to the trinity of what is known as the Eight Trigrams which symbolize the attributes of all the physical and cosmic conditions on Earth and correlate with the Eight Directions of the Medicine Wheel.

The trigrams are the development of the yang/yin symbology from a two-line to a three-line representation. The two lines represent the duality in Nature – the visible and invisible, the light and darkness, hot and cold – and the four ways the forces can come together.

The third line represents the individual, who combines within her- or himself both the visible and the invisible, the conscious and the unconscious, the physical and spiritual, and stands between Heaven and Earth.

Now there are only eight ways this trinity can be expressed:

1	2	3	4	5	6	7	8
Three yang	Yin above yang	Yin in middle of yang	Two yin above yang	Yin at bottom of yang	Yang in middle of yin	Yang above yin	Three yin
All light	light more than dark	Dark inside light	Light less than dark	Light more than dark	Light inside dark	Dark more than light	All Dark

These eight trigrams can be used to represent all the principal physical and spiritual conditions on Earth. No one knows who devised them, but according to ancient legends they were derived from Nature. They were in use before the six-line symbols of the oriental *I Ching*, or 'Book of Changes', appeared under Fu Hsi, the First Emperor of China, nearly 5,000 years ago, and made use of the trigrams by pairing them into hexagrams with sixty-four (8x8) possible combinations.

The I Ching (pronounced Yee Jing) is sometimes falsely described as a fortune-telling system, but it is no such thing. It is an oracle of profound mystical writings, packed with practical wisdom, and has been consulted in the Orient for thousands of years as a guide and an adviser in facing the changes and challenges of everyday life, though it was hardly known in the West until the first half of the twentieth century.

The Tai Chi emblem depicted earlier in Figure 15 is a symbol of the Moon placed over that of the Sun to represent the principle of change and duality. The 'I' (Yee) means 'changes' and the 'Ching' (Jing) means book or system. So I Ching means the Book or System of Changes. The system is the co-ordinates produced through a pairing of the eight trigrams.

Selection of a six-line hexagram is made in according with the I Ching's method of enquiry, using yarrow sticks or coins, but it is simply a mechanical way of tapping into the unconscious mind. The hexagram arrived at when a question is put is said to reveal a person's present state of mind and, therefore, what must follow is predictable because the unconscious mind will act to bring about what has been impressed upon it unless the state of mind is changed or modified.

The Oracle may warn of possible difficulties and advise on how to establish a state of harmony and balance between the conscious and unconscious and between the outer and inner lives. The solution, however, rests with the enquirer, who is regarded, as with American Indian spirituality, as having responsibility for his own life.

The I Ching was not, of course, an integral part of the Medicine Wheel. Native Americans of old had no books and their writing was in the form of pictograms and not words, but the I Ching was know by travelling shamans who gleaned knowledge from sources beyond their own tribal traditions. The Mayan Indian had a numerical system, using dots and bars, some of whose combinations looked very similar to I Ching symbols and trigrams and this was used to relate the conscious with the unconscious, the outer with the inner, the physical with the spiritual.

The I Ching is mentioned in this book for two principal reasons. First, its concept of the yang and yin duality in Nature expresses perhaps more clearly to the Western mind the spiritual sexuality principle of the Indian. Second, the Medicine Wheel and the I Ching developed from the same ancient source and are compatible and complementary.

The I Ching can be used in partnership with Earth Medicine since it is constructed in accordance with similar principles to those of the Medicine Wheel. In other words, although Earth Medicine is primarily an analytical system, the I Ching is its natural extension into an Oracle.

The Eight Trigrams of the I Ching can be arranged on the Eight Directions of the Medicine Wheel as show in Figure 38.

This differs from the traditional arrangements to be found in various books on the circular I Ching, but it represents the I Ching's correlation with Medicine Wheel teachings, and we shall look at this further in Part Three to see how it can be put to *practical* use.

I have endeavoured to indicate that the Medicine Wheel correlates with all other cultures of antiquity – with the circular I Ching of the East, with the zodiac of the West, and with the Wheel of the Year of the Caucasian peoples of the North, of Britain, northern Europe and Scandinavia. The Medicine Wheel may thus be seen as a catalyst of ancient wisdom and a means of reclaiming much of the lost esoteric knowledge of the past.

Since Earth Medicine is a part of that 'lost' knowledge and relates to the Medicine Wheel, to other circular philosophies, and to the Wheel of the Year of ancient Caucasian cultures, it is presented in chart form on the following pages along the lines of a Web.

The Web was an ancient symbolic device used by Caucasian shamans in olden times to explain and describe the interwoven, interconnecting and interacting web of energy that surrounds us and forms what we regard as reality, and is thus of particular significance.

The Web mandala is intended to emphasize the concept that everything is connected and that what we perceive in the world of ordinary reality is in actuality energy forms. Everything has a bio-plasmic energy field and is connected with other energy fields by veins of flowing energy frequencies like strands of a spider's web. Touch one and all are in some way affected.

Nothing, therefore, exists in isolation. Everything is interconnected and interrelated within a vast cosmic reservoir of pulsating energy with access to the Source that is both at the centre of all things and is that in which all things exist.

Further, we as individuals are not only the 'weavers' of our own 'Web' – our own 'little' universe – but we are also the Web itself.

That is a key to the ancient wisdom. That is at the essence of Medicine Wheel teachings. That is the 'secret' of acquiring an understanding of all the 'mysteries'.

Trigram	I Ching image	Position on the Web
1 Ch'ien	Heaven	This is placed in the north-east which is the direction of beginnings – the beginning of spring and the year.
2 Tui	Lake	This is allocated to the south-east. The Lake is associated with joy, pleasure and openness, so the position of the Summer Solstice on the Wheel expresses the time when people get out into the open and experience the joy and pleasure of hot days in the Sun.
3 Li	Fire	This is placed in the East, which in Medicine cosmology is the direction for elemental Fire. The I Ching describes this element as 'the *clinging* Fire', which describes another of its characteristics.
4 Chen	Thunder	Thunder changes the atmosphere and is sudden and expansive. It is allocated to the south-west.
5 Sun	Wind	This is placed in the North, the direction for elemental Air. In the I Ching it is described as 'the gentle wind that penetrates'. Since the North is also associated with the mind and the intellect, its relevance here is clear.
6 Kan	Water	This is placed in the direction for elemental Water in the South.
7 Ken	Mountain	This is allocated to the north-west and is sometimes described as 'keeping still'. The north-west is thus appropriate since it positions the Winter Solstice on the Web – the dead of winter.
8 K'un	Earth	Again, following the positioning of the Elements on the Web, this is assigned the direction for elemental Earth in the West. It is described as 'gentle, yielding and nurturing'.

It is the realization of that which can put us back into harmony with Nature, with the Earth, and with ourselves – and, of course, with one another.

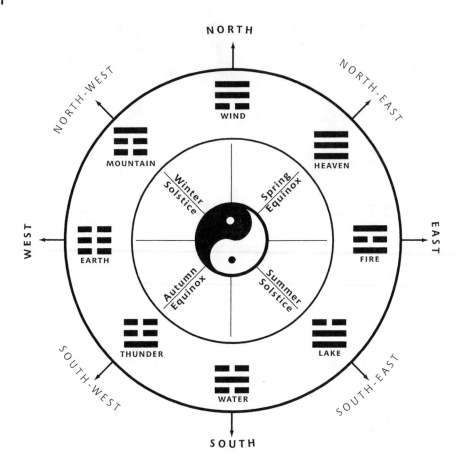

Figure 38. The eight Trigrams and eight Directions in the Northern Hemisphere

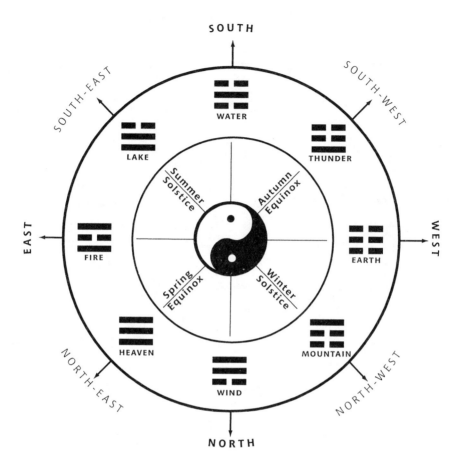

Figure 38(a). The eight Trigrams and eight Directions in the Southern Hemisphere

PART TWO

The Analysis

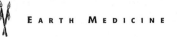

Look To The Earth

Look to the Earth
And to the Skies
The Sun, the Moon, and to the stars
You who would be wise.
For they contain the full measure of man
The height, the breadth, the depth, the span
Of his entirety.

Look to the Earth
And to the skies
And watch them turn
Like pages of a holy book
But one untouched by human hand
You who would be wise.

Look to the Earth
And to the skies
For in that which can be seen Without
Can true knowledge come
Of unseen mysteries that lie Within
To you who would be wise.

Look to the Earth
And to the skies
In Spring and Summer
Winter and in the Fall.
Watch life begin, unfold, then fade and die
To rise anew
Time and again for Time Untold
You who would be wise.

Look to the Earth
And to the skies
And in your looking, learn this mystery:
That you who look to the Earth
And to the skies
Shall be given eyes to see
Shall be given eyes
To make you wise
Eternally.

Kenneth Meadows, 1988

Introduction to Part Two

IF YOU HAVE READ PART ONE OF THIS BOOK THOUGHTFULLY, YOU will have grasped the basic principles of Earth Medicine and gained an insight into American Indian spirituality that will enable you to become attuned to its sensitivities.

From the chapters dealing with the solar, lunar and earth influences and the directional and elemental forces, you will have gleaned an awareness of the foundational essences from which your personality was formed.

In Part Two, a section is devoted to each of the twelve birth totems of Earth Medicine and the twelve personality expressions through which life is perceived and experienced. In the section dealing with your own birth totem, you will find indications concerning your personality characteristics, your tendencies and your potentials, and also a suggestion of the possible Quest and Life Path of your Real Self – the inner 'hidden' you – to help you come to a realization that your life does, indeed, have purpose.

Of course, since the information given in each section will apply equally to all people born within its time-period of approximately thirty days, these can be only broad and general indications, but none the less they should prove helpful enough. Of course, not everyone born in the same section of time will have identical personalities and see things in exactly the same way. Every individual is different. Indeed, every individual is unique and developing in their own way. But people who are born in the same Earth Influence period share certain broad characteristics and attitudes just as people born in a particular region of a country share its local dialect.

We are all citizens of the world, but we are not all alike. There are pronounced differences, like the colour of skin, and racial and cultural attitudes. Further distinctions are determined by the country of our birth. For instance, a person born in the United Kingdom and a person born in the United States will both speak English, but there will be differences in the way the language is spoken, and certain words will not even have the same meaning. Each will approach life from different social and cultural backgrounds which will influence the way they interpret life.

Even when people have similar character traits and qualities, they may express them differently, but none the less there will be a broad but distinctive behaviour pattern and it is this that each birth totem section will indicate.

As in Nature, the energies we are examining here are not static and fixed. They are flowing and in constant motion. American Indians likened this flow to the tides of the Moon. The Moon's energies build up as the surface of its reflected light increases and reach their peak at the Full Moon. Then they diminish as the Moon wanes and less of the surface is lit. So with humans there are similar modes of expression of the character traits and qualities and these will be examined.

A further factor is that energies can be projected either positively or negatively. Every character trait has a positive polarity – a constructive aspect – and a negative polarity, or adverse aspect, and each contains the seed of its own opposite in accordance with the law of duality, yang and yin. So the person who is domineering and dictatorial is expressing the negative aspects of the protective and nurturing. Someone who is manipulative and underhand is expressing the negative polarity of the helpful and unassuming. Similarly, a person who is indecisive and selfish is displaying the negative aspects of one who is dependable and caring.

The sections in Part Two are also of especial help in understanding other people – your loved ones, members of your family, friends, colleagues and associates.

Naturally, most readers will want to read the section concerning themselves and those of their loved ones first, but in order to obtain the maximum benefit the whole of Part Two should be read thoroughly because each section contains not only a penetrating insight into the different streams of personality, but also important elements of the 'hidden' teachings of American Indians and these apply to everyone and not just those whose birthdays occur during the time being dealt with.

Part Three suggests how you can achieve a finer tuning of the system through practical application of the principles of Earth Medicine. It also shows how to move around the Web gathering qualities you need and correcting your own recognized imbalances. And it includes methods of obtaining *intuitive* knowledge, knowledge that is personal to you, and relevant to the circumstances of your life.

Of course, the ultimate value of any self-help, self-development system, comes from its personal application. In Earth Medicine that comes from putting your totems to work for you.

So far you have been introduced to three personal totems. You have a birth or animal totem – Falcon, Beaver, Deer, Woodpecker, Salmon, Brown Bear, Crow, Snake, Owl, Goose, Otter or Wolf, depending on the time of the year of your birthday – a directional totem (either Eagle, Mouse, Grizzly or Buffalo) and an elemental totem (Hawk, Frog, Turtle or Butterfly).

In working through your section you will acquire other totems. Remember, these totems are *symbolic* representations of intangible forces and qualities, and therefore helpful mental tools and memory aids to enable you to systematize information and to associate ideas. But they can become much more than that if you want Earth Medicine to really *work* for you.

Your totems can become active *helpers* in the development of your intuitive senses for they can act as connectors to the different levels with which they are associated. To use an analogy, they are like the functional keys of a personal computer which can key you in to a whole range of information and also provide you with access to the performance of certain tasks.

The information thus obtained is *intuitive* knowledge because it comes not from a book or a computer program but from within the self. It is an *insight* – an inner 'see-ing' – that goes beyond the process of reasoning things out. It is *illumination* that lies beyond the intellect and once obtained becomes truth that is personal to you.

Each section in Part Two is really a charting device. Its purpose is to enable you to see yourself more clearly and to recognize how you are affected by the energies manifesting in your life. You will then be better able to work with them and to live up to your full potential.

Each section is arranged in the following sequence:

1. *Birth month*: This gives the starting and ending dates of the approximate thirty-day time-period.

2. *Earth influence*: The prime influence that affects the time-period is indicated succinctly in the way Nature usually expresses itself during that part of the yearly cycle, e.g. the *Awakening* Time (21 March – 19 April), when Nature appears to awaken from its winter rest and springs into new life: the *Growing* Time (20 April – 20 May), when vegetation puts down roots and shows rapid growth above the surface of the soil; and *Long Days* Time (21 June – 21 July), the period of long days and short nights, and the *Blustery Winds* Time (19 February – 20 March), the period of strong winds and gales. What is being examined, though, is not the effect of *physical* forces

but of the non-physical essences that activate and ensoul all material manifestation. The Earth influence encapsulates those essences and forces.

3. *Solar influence*: This indicates the seasonal character of the solar energies, whether they are waxing or waning, and how they affect the human condition. The related Sun sign in Sun astrology is indicated so that you may refer to correlated information in this area of the ancient sciences.

4. *Influencing wind*: The appropriate directional power is identified and its fundamental and possible effect examined.

5. *Influencing elements*: The elemental forces influencing the personality are examined in both their directional and cyclical modes, and the possible effect on the personality is discussed.

6. *Elemental clan*: The Elemental Clan – Earth, Water, Air, Fire – to which the individual is related through birth in a particular time-period is examined and its implications discussed.

7–10. *Totems*: The birth totem (animal), and plant, mineral and polarity totems are identified and their purpose, meaning and value in interpreting tendencies are discussed in detail.

11. *Personality expression*: This is a detailed analysis of how people born under a particular Earth influence express themselves to others, and of core characteristics and likely tendencies. It indicates how the personality is likely to express itself it childhood, and as an adult, and as a parent. The potentialities and possible talents are also given, together with an indication of the vocational areas in which job satisfaction is likely to be found.

12. *Romance and sex*: The probable romantic outlook is assessed, together with the possible sexual attitude. The most likely compatibilities between the sexes are also given.

13. *Health*: A summary of likely health tendencies and possible problem areas.

14. *Affinity colour*: The affinity colour of the birth totem is given and its significance explained. This information provides a useful introduction to the subject of colour harmonics and colour therapy.

15. *Advantageous times*: The month, day and times in the day when the cosmic energies harmonize to provide the most likely advantageous period for personal development.

16. *Outward aim and inner desire*: The outward (conscious) aim is the direction that life appears to be headed in and the impression that is

being given to others; the inner (subconscious) desire is the 'hidden' tendency. Both are analysed.

17. *Spiritual alchemy*: An assessment of the extrovert (masculine) and introvert (feminine) tendencies within the fundamental personality of the relevant Earth influence and where to look to balance the inner dynamics.

18. *Life challenges*: Experiences that are likely to be encountered frequently, and the lessons they are there to teach. They are the opportunities to strengthen character through karmic programming.

19. *Life-path and primary function*: Where to find the true purpose of your life.

20. *Influencing I Ching trigram*: The relevant I Ching trigram in accordance with the energies flowing in the Earth Influence period. Knowledge of this is helpful in developing an extension into mystical counselling.

21. *How to cope with people of this birth totem*: If you are studying a section in order to understand more about someone you know, this gives a brief outline on how best to deal with them.

Note Each subsection is prefixed with the section number followed by the subsection number; e.g. 1.6 is section 1 (Awakening Time, Falcon) subsection 6 (elemental clan); 8.4 is section 8 (Frost Time, Snake) subsection 4 (influencing wind). This is to make cross-referencing and comparisons quick and easy.

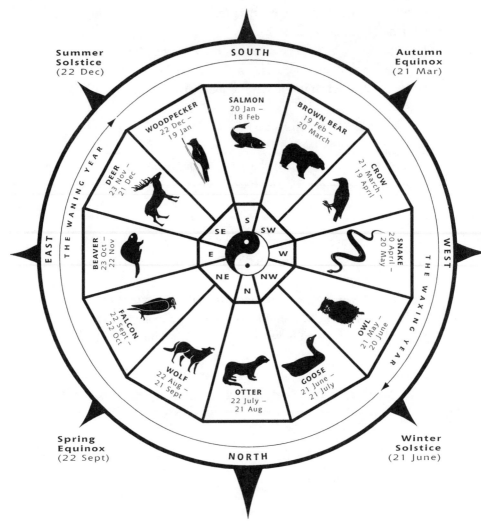

Figure 38(b). The Earth Medicine Web for the Southern hemisphere

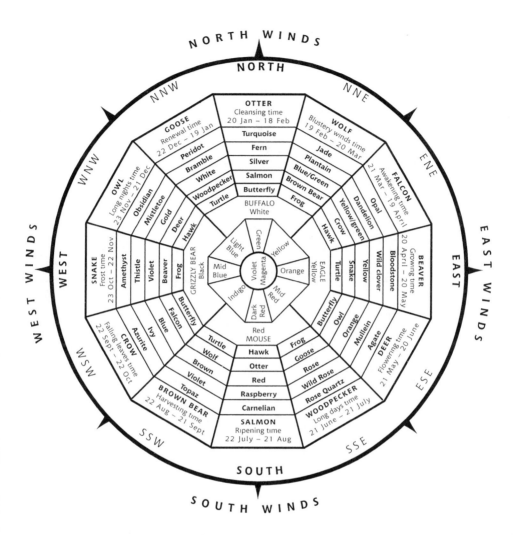

Figure 39. The Earth Medicine Web for the Northern hemisphere

Falcon

SUMMARY

Birth dates:	21 March – 19 April (22 September – 22 October in the Southern hemisphere).
Earth influence:	The Awakening Time.
Influencing wind:	The East Winds. *Totem:* Eagle.
Direction:	North-east.
Predominant element:	Fire.
Elemental clan:	Hawk (Fire) Clan. *Function:* to initiate.
Birth and animal totem:	Falcon.
Plant totem:	Dandelion.
Mineral totem:	Opal.
Polarity totem:	Crow.
Affinity colour:	Yellow/green.
Personality:	Active. Forceful. Impetuous.
Feelings:	Quickly aroused.
Intention:	Activity – new beginnings.
Nature:	Impulsive.
Positive traits:	Enterprising. Pioneering. Adventurous. Affable.
Negative traits:	Selfish. Egotistical. Impatient. Ostentatious.
Sex-drive:	Easily aroused. Quick, fiery and passionate.
Compatibilities:	Salmon and Owls.
Conscious aim:	To initiate and lead.
Subconscious desire:	Knowledge through personal experience.
Life-path:	Establishment of individuality through discernment.
I Ching trigram:	☰ Ch'ien. Heaven. Success through effort.
Spiritual alchemy:	Yang predominates.
Must cultivate:	Patience. Persistence. Compassion.
Must avoid:	Vanity. Conceit. Intolerance.
Starting totems:	Falcon. Eagle. Hawk. Dandelion. Opal. Crow.

1. Falcon

1.1 BIRTH MONTH: 21 March – 19 April

1.2 EARTH INFLUENCE: The Awakening Time

The Awakening Time is the first of the three cycles of spring and begins the growth-and-illumination cycle of the East at the Spring Equinox on 21 March.

People born between 21 March and 19 April enter Earth life at the time of the yearly cycle when that which has been lying dormant and within the darkness of the Earth during winter is waking into new life. Those born at this time express the newness of the life-energy that requires the patient nurturing of loving care to being it into full blossom.

These human 'buddings' are like the seeds that push up their first shoots out of the soil in springtime, and the buds that burst into life on trees and plants – full of exuberant energy, but not yet fully aware of the world beyond themselves.

They are being driven by an urge to demonstrate their existence as individuals. What they will need to come to recognize is that they are not alone, and that the ideas that seem to spring so readily from their minds contain only *potential* and require the help and co-operation of others to bring them to the maturity of practical reality.

The Awakening Time brings energy for speedy growth and for change, for this is one of the most rapid periods of growth in the Earth's yearly cycle. So those born in the Awakening Time are here to develop rapidly and in so doing learn the lesson of all growing things – adaptability. For part of their life's purpose is the learning of patience and persistence, and especially adaptability, without compromising on ideals and principles.

The Awakening Time begins at the Spring Equinox, which marks the arrival of spring when the Earth Mother brings forth new life that has lain within her womb during the winter. It is the time of the promised rebirth which was implicit in death. It is the resurrection into new life of that which appeared to be dead and to have vanished for ever into invisibility. Its message is evident everywhere around – in the blush of green leaves on the trees, in the springiness of the grass beneath the feet, in the budding plants, and in the blossoming of the spring flowers that open their hearts to shout their message of joy and wonder.

It is a message not just of awakening, but of reawakening, for it is the time of re-becoming.

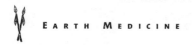

With it come the fresh spring winds that enrich the air with new oxygen and blow into our lives giving us the vigour to clear out the clutter of debris that has accumulated over the winter. It is the time for a new spring outfit of clothes to brighten us and to help us to sense our renewal.

1.3 SOLAR INFLUENCES

This is the beginning of the spring season when the Solar energies are waxing and gaining strength and bringing new life into manifestation. So people of this month will want to project themselves into the world of practical experience with enthusiasm and to look for opportunities to display their creativity. They will seek mental exploration and consideration of moral issues.

The temperament might be described as warming. There may be an almost shy uncertainty that might be mistaken for aloofness and even indifference. But behind it, at the core, is deep affection which comes forth only through gentle arousal.

The related Sun sign is Aries.

1.4 INFLUENCING WIND: The East Winds
DIRECTION: North-East

Since the East Winds of Spring tempt people out into the open after their long periods spent indoors during winter, a quality associated with the East winds is open-mindedness. So the need for open-mindedness is likely to be evident in the lives of those born in the Awakening Time. When they maintain an open mind towards a situation with which they are confronted, they will be in harmony with the energies that influence them, but should they adopt a stubborn or dogmatic attitude and close their minds, the flow of energies will be blocked and create obstructions and difficulties for them.

As the East winds come from the direction of the dawn and the rising sun, they are also associated with awakening, of coming into a new awareness as illumination begins to reveal that which was once hidden or obscured. People of this time will feel the urge for illumination in all areas of their life; the need to see things more clearly, why they are as they are, and how things work out.

People born in the Awakening Time are affected by the directional power of the East – one might describe it as the spirit or intelligence of the East – whose energies stimulate the desire to start new projects, to be involved in new challenges, and to make fresh beginnings.

A totem that helped the Indians to relate more readily to such an intangible spiritual force, and the totem that was used by many tribes as a meaningful symbol of the East, was the *eagle*.

Characteristic of the eagle is its ability to see great distances, and far-sightedness was considered an important quality of the East. It is of particular relevance to people born in the Awakening Time for it stresses the importance of not being hurried into a situation because of any apparent immediate advantages and the need to look ahead and to consider the long-term consequences of any proposed action.

Since the power of the East influence is primarily with the spirit, Awakening Time folk are likely to be attracted to interests which emphasize spiritual considerations or moral or ethical issues. They will be drawn into experiences which are intended to bring their attention to the relevance of principles.

1.5 INFLUENCING ELEMENT: **Fire**

Elemental Fire is associated with the spiritual plane of existence which is sensed not with the eyes or the ears, nor by touch, but with the heart. It is experienced through love – not the love of self-indulgence, but the love that is a giving of oneself. This is one of the great realizations for Awakening Time people to come to experience in their lives.

Awakening Time folk are influenced by the power of elemental Fire, and it is this energy that is evident in their burning enthusiasm for the things that attract them, and – if they do not learn to control it – the energy behind their impulsiveness and fiery temperament when provoked.

People of this time seem full of energy and always on the go, and it is elemental Fire that is their energizer and driving power. In addition, they will be creative, enthusiastic, versatile and extroverted, all of which are expressions of the qualities of elemental Fire.

1.6 ELEMENTAL CLAN: **Hawk Clan**

The hawk is a large and magnificent bird of prey which is spectacular in its flight. The red hawk was venerated by many Indian tribes and its feathers were treasured and used in ceremonials, especially for healing. It was often associated with the phoenix, the mythical firebird which arose out of its own burning ashes and was symbolic of radiant energy, the blazing of new trails, the flash of intuition, and the thunder of sudden change.

The elemental clan gives an indication of the principal function of those who belong to it – the fundamental contribution of the people who comprise it to the rest of the tribe or community. The Hawk Clan can be considered the thinkers, inspirers and leaders. Those born in the Awakening Time are the 'starters' – the pioneers who lead the way ahead for others. They are the ones who start new activity and set it in motion from the heat of their own inner fire.

Awakening Time people look around for new things to be involved in, and begin new projects for others to build on. They light new fires for others to keep alight. They have an intuitive sense which, like lightning, comes in sudden flashes of illumination, but they need to look for guidance from people of other Times in the Clan on how to develop this intuitive sense, for it can often provide the insight they need when faced with important decisions.

Since elemental Fire is exerting its influence both directionally and cyclically, they must guard against becoming too intense about the way they express their energies and live their lives, otherwise they run the risk of burning themselves out eventually.

1.7 BIRTH AND ANIMAL TOTEM: Falcon

There are many species of falcon, but all have long, pointed wings and long tails and a large head and neck in proportion to body size. Falcons are not nesters, like hawks, but lay their eggs on ledges or in the disused nests of other birds. Falcons are spectacular in flight, taking their prey after high-speed swoops, often from great heights.

The heavily built and beautifully proportioned prairie falcon (*Falco mexicanus*) was a popular totem among some tribes and so was the American kestrel (*Falco sparverius*). In Europe the possible equivalent is the common kestrel (*Falco tinnunculus*), which is the best-known falcon.

The kestrel is one of the most handsome birds of prey, and one of the most helpful to humans because it feeds on insects such as grasshoppers and beetles that can be quite destructive to crops. And although it is fierce, it can also be gentle, and is a bird that can be trained. Significantly, it was a favourite bird used in the ancient pastime of falconry throughout Europe.

The kestrel has a grey head and a grey, fan-like tail with a black band at the edge. Its back is chestnut brown. Like all falcons, it has a hooked beak and taloned feet. Kestrels are a joy to watch in flight as they circle and soar and then swoop at great speed, sometimes from a considerable height, to take their prey. They frequently hover before pouncing, with wings flapping vigorously and tail fanned out.

Awakening Time people, like their totem, like to spread their wings. They, too, are hunters, but their prey is a new idea, a new experience, new places to visit, or new things to do. They, too, are fearless when going after the things they want.

As the falcon is able to rise to great heights, so do people of this totem, for they have high ideals. They sometimes, though, lack the patience to see things through and can be all too easily distracted.

Falcon people are good starters, but not such good stayers and finishers. Part of their life-purpose is, in fact, to learn to balance their energies by nurturing a situation and staying with it long enough to bring it to fruition.

Falcon people lack the concentration to stay long enough with a particular situation to derive the fullest benefit from it, and quickly tire of what they have begun, moving on to the next attraction that catches their eye. Though they enter every new challenge with enthusiasm, they often lack the staying power that brings the fullest rewards. Persistence is thus a quality anyone born in this time needs to develop.

Another lesson that people of the Awakening Time are learning from life is that the way to resolve the kind of problem which repeatedly confronts them is not to search elsewhere for the solution. The solution is to be found in the experience of the problem itself.

1.8 PLANT TOTEM: Dandelion

The plant totem of Falcon people is the dandelion (*Taraxacum officinale*), a perennial found almost everywhere on grassland and wasteland and on banks through North America and Europe. In cultivated areas it is considered to be something of a nuisance.

Its broad-bladed leaves grow out from the milky taproot in rosettes around long, hollow stalks, and have jagged, irregular, tooth-like edges. Indeed, it is this feature which gave the plant its English name, for the word 'Dandelion' is a corruption of the French for 'lion's tooth' – *dent-de-lion*. The yellow flower-heads are made up of some 200 different florets which close up at night or in dull weather.

All parts of the plant can be used medicinally – roots, leaves and flowers.

The dandelion is also called the puffball or blowball because of its familiar cluster of seeds which succeed the flower and have fluffy, down-like tufts which carry the seeds like a parachute in the wind. The seeds will grow almost anywhere they land.

Falcon people are like their dandelion totem – easily blown from one place to another, from one idea to the next, and flying into things without taking the time to look them over. At the same time they need to be useful and can take root anywhere.

Though it is rated as a nuisance by gardeners and cultivators of the soil, Dandelion is full of character and a treasure-house of beneficial properties. For instance, its root affects all forms of secretion and excretion from the human body. It promotes the formation of bile and helps remove poisons from the body, so it acts as a tonic and a stimulant.

The root can be dried and used as a caffeine-free coffee substitute for it has a taste similar to instant coffee. As a herbal remedy, it is especially helpful in dealing with liver problems, and helps to balance the blood sugar.

Dandelion leaves are healthful as salad greens for they are rich in vitamin A, and also contain vitamins B, C and G as well as essential minerals like calcium, iron, phosphorus and sodium which help to purify the blood.

Like their plant totem, Falcon people have a tendency to open up, not only to new ideas and new projects in which they become involved, but also to the minds of people with whom they come into contact.

Their forthrightness also tends to act as a purgative of things and concepts that have served their purpose and are no longer of continuing value, for although others may not appreciate Falcons' bluntness and directness in speaking their mind, it often stimulates them into taking action in those apparently sensitive areas and to eliminate what is no longer necessary.

Falcon people may find much value themselves in the soothing and healing properties of their plant totem.

1.9 MINERAL TOTEM: Opal

The mineral totem of Falcons is the opal – a glassy, translucent stone which is a non-crystalline form of quartz. The common opal is milky white, but there are forms that are black and a greenish-yellow, and another called fire opal which has luminous reds and purples in it.

Opal comes from hot places and where there is pressure – like the cavities of volcanic rock or near hot springs. So it is a stone that is used to coping with heat and withstanding pressure and consequently can be of particular help to those who find themselves under emotional pressure or undergoing fiery trials.

Opal is composed of silicone dioxide, which the ancients regarded as 'solidified cosmic light'. It is found wherever there is a surging upward towards the light. Silica is found in the nodes of the stalks of grasses and cereals and enables the hollow stems to stand erect. It is in the cartilage of the intervertebral disc of the spine. Silica is contained also in the lens of the eye and is thus concerned with clarity. So the opal is linked with the striving upwards of the idealist and the quest for clarity and truth – again signs of the Falcon personality.

Opal has a strong reflective nature and contains cosmic rays that amplify the traits of the human being that holds it. So it will strengthen the traits of its wearer, whether positive or negative, and since it is so sensitive to changes of vibrations it is a stone to be held rather than worn.

Falcon people have an inquisitive nature and opals will enhance the ability to look into things and so help in seeing into them rather more deeply.

Some tribes held the fire opal in high regard and because opal contains a proportion of water, the fire opal was sometimes referred to as 'the fire that spreads like water'. I was told that the stone is therefore helpful to anyone who is encountering the 'fire that springs from the water of the emotions'. Falcon people will encounter plenty of life-experiences whose purpose is to teach them mastery of their emotions and fire opal is a stone with great harmonizing powers on an emotional level and is especially beneficial in dispersing emotional negativity.

Opal is a stone of the idealist whose quest for truth springs from the heart rather than the intellect.

1.10 POLARITY TOTEM: Crow

The complementary totem for Falcons is the Crow (22 September – 22 October). Like their totem, Crow people are generally adaptable, fast movers, but down-to-earth. Though the birds are considered something of a nuisance to farmers, American Indians regarded them as creatures of balance since they served a vital purpose in the ecology as scavengers of things that had been discarded and thus needed to be disposed of. There are many species of crow, of which the raven is the largest. The raven builds its nest on the tops of trees or in high places and though it soars to great heights, spends much time on the land from which it feeds. The Indian interpreted this as combining the energies of the sky (Air) with the land (Earth) and thus a indication of the need to express ideas in the world of practical reality.

So Crow, as a polarity totem, is stressing to Falcon that the pursuit of self-interest inherent in the Falcon requires careful balance if it is not to soar off into the extremes of fanaticism.

As Falcon is an expression of the individual, so its polarity, Crow, which prefers groups or flocks, is an expression of grouping or community. So for balance Falcons should look to service to a group, and to develop a sense of loyalty and commitment to a community. In other words, the message of Crow is that idealism, to be of any true value, needs to be balanced with practical, down-to-earth endeavour that brings benefit to others as well as to the self.

Falcon people will find fulfilment when they seek opportunities to balance individualistic pursuits with service to others in *practical* ways. Crow is thus directing Falcons to have their feet planted firmly on the ground and to bring down to Earth the things that they come to learn in the sky.

1.11 PERSONALITY EXPRESSION
Adult

Like the new shoots of spring, those born in the Awakening Time are 'pushers', even hustling others into participating in their schemes, only to lose interest when a new project is under way and they are off again pushing a new interest.

Extroverted, exuberant, restless, enterprising, energetic Falcon seems designed for *action*. Falcon people are the initiators, but with an impulsiveness that makes them prone to making hasty judgements which they may later come to regret.

Their optimistic nature and determined will, however, enable them to overcome disappointment and failure and to rise above any adversity.

They have a strong sense of independence which gives them a 'go-it-alone' attitude if partners or colleagues do not respond readily to their ideas. They have an active imagination which, coupled with an infectious enthusiasm, inclines them to exaggerate and to fantasize.

Falcons are not the world's best diplomats. Indeed, their frankness and their tendency to 'speak their minds' makes them prone to tactlessness that can sometimes put them in dire predicaments.

Since Falcons are strongly influenced by the element of Fire, as we have seen, their essential nature is energetic and enthusiastic, though impulsive and easily aroused. The Falcon person's flame burns fiercely, but for only a short while, so they have to learn how to control it.

Falcons must guard against being so carried away by their own sense of self-importance that they become blinded by conceit and vanity. They tend to live for the moment, easily cutting themselves off from the past, and disregarding future consequences. To the Falcon it is the present that counts.

Positive traits: Pioneering. Adventurous. Enterprising. Courageous. Energetic. Affable.

Negative traits: Selfish. Egotistical. Impulsive. Impatient. Quick-tempered. Ostentatious.

Vocational possibilities: Acting. Adventurous occupations. Dentistry. Electronics. Engineering. Firefighting. Hairdressing. Jewellery-making. Journalism. The Armed Forces. Professional sports. Stenography. Surgery.

Child

The infant Falcon starts to walk sooner than most children, but this readiness in finding its feet makes it accident-prone and parents need to guard against injuries through falling and bumping into things.

Falcon infants are affectionate and loveable, but quite demanding, and their fiery nature is soon in evidence in their quickness of temper when their demands are thwarted. Their impatience, too, shows quite early in their unwillingness to wait. They want their sweets *now* – a characteristic which stays with them throughout life unless tamed.

The Falcon child needs to be gently disciplined from an early age, otherwise it will suffer more painfully in adulthood when it comes up against authority and competition, but handled harshly it is likely to develop a mean streak.

Falcon children will relish stories told to them, and as they grow older develop a love for the written word. They are bright, but often reluctant to put real effort into their school work, so they need encouragement and incentive. Falcon children seem to respond to praise and to challenge rather than punishment, and regard criticism as an attack and react to it adversely.

As children, Falcons need to be kept busy and active, otherwise their idle hands will find mischief, but they require plenty of sleep in order to renew their energies. Sensibly and affectionately handled, the Falcon child will live up to what is expected of it.

Parent

Although Falcon parents tend to be rather disciplinarian, they generally raise offspring who develop a sense of independence as they mature.

The Falcon male makes a proud and devoted father, though he may be resentful if his wife demotes him to second place in her affections. He can be dogmatic and even dictatorial as the children get into their teens, especially about their choice of career, or even of friends.

The Falcon mother is caring, but not to the point of fussing over her children or of being over-protective. Her imaginativeness helps her to create an enjoyable fantasy world for her children.

1.12 ROMANCE AND SEX

The imagination plays an important part in romance for the Falcon person as well as in other areas of life. The Falcon male is looking for a story-book romance and for a 'princess' to be his one true love. He usually makes a faithful lover, though he wants his own way in marriage. The female Falcon will tend to put her lover on a pedestal and expect rather too much of him. Both male and female Falcons have a possessive nature and a jealous streak as well as a temper that can be hurtful to their partner.

The male Falcon can be a whirlwind lover and whisk a girl off her feet with the ardour of his attention, but he does tend to be rather chauvinist. He can be flirtatious for it stimulates his ego, but woe betide the man who makes eyes at his partner. His attitude will be very much 'She belongs to me!'

The female Falcon can be alluring, with a charisma that is attractive and seductive, but her outspokenness, frankness and sudden tantrums can be a big turn-off. She has a tendency to be bossy, and in marriage is likely to be the one to wear the trousers. She is, however, a romantic and will respond to affection with a tender and generous heart.

Falcons like sweet words for it elevates their sense of self-importance, but they need to beware of falling prey to the smooth talker.

Falcon men and women are easily turned on, and make fiery and passionate lovers, but their love-making is usually brief and short-lived. In sexual matters, as in other areas of their lives, they need to learn patience and to consider the needs of their partners and not just their own.

Compatibilities: Falcons are compatible with Salmon and Owls (those born between 21 July and 21 August, and 23 November and 21 December).

Spiritual sexuality: (+) The basic spiritual sexuality of Falcons is masculine, but this is not concerned with gender. It means that Falcons are usually active, energetic and extroverted. They are the initiators. In physical relationships they are likely to be fiery and impulsive.

1.13 HEALTH

The Awakening Time is related to the area of the head in the physical body
and to the brain of the internal body. It also has an influence on the glands
which pump adrenalin into the bloodstream. Falcons may be prone to
health problems in these areas – especially headaches and migraines and
nervous disorders resulting from stress. These are warning signs of the
need to relax and be less intense. Stress and nervous disorders can be
caused by trying to do too much, or when the urge to get things done
becomes frustrated, or emotionally when there is a feeling of not doing
enough. Falcons must learn from Nature, for Nature is not all activity, but
alternates between action and rest.

As Fire people, Falcons are susceptible, too, to high blood-pressure and
to complaints that arise suddenly.

1.14 AFFINITY COLOUR: Yellow/green

The affinity colour combination of Falcon is yellow changing to green.
Yellow is a cheerful colour for it is the colour of sunshine which comes
from the East as a refined expression of creativity. It is the colour
associated with the intellect and expresses a need for constant stimulation
and activity.

Green is the colour of Nature and of growing things – of balance in the
midst of continual change. It is associated with the Creative Fire that
contained within it the Water of Life and the means to enable vegetation to
spring forth in order that life could be sustained.

Yellow/green signifies an aspect of being between the mental and the
material and which promotes both mental and physical digestion. This
colour combination stimulates a need for recognition and popularity. It is
the colour of a personality that seeks to impress.

1.15 ADVANTAGEOUS TIMES

Best months of the year for Falcon people are from 21 March to 19 April, 22
July to 21 August, and 23 October to 21 December.
Best day of the week is Tuesday.
Best times of the day are from 3 p.m. to 5 p.m.

Falcons are at their brightest in the early morning, which is their best
time for finding inspiration. The more routine work is best left for the
afternoon when the creative and inspirational energies dip, and it is more
productive to undertake the more 'mechanical' chores. The early evening is
best for relaxation and to recharge the batteries.

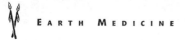

1.16 OUTWARD (CONSCIOUS) AIM AND INNER (SUBCONSCIOUS) DESIRE

The conscious aim of the Falcon is to initiate and to lead and to start new things. Since Falcons seek self-expression, they will show a strong tendency to want their own way in any project in which they become involved. This urge may be so powerful that they are prone to react childishly if their ideas are challenged, or if they can't have their own way for whatever reason.

The desire of the Falcon's inner self is to come to *know* through personal experience. Falcon people are self-orientated and self-motivated because of this inner drive to experience things for themselves. Falcons will rise to challenges of all kinds in pursuit of whatever goal happens to have captured their interest at the time. What they are seeking is the knowledge that comes from personal experience.

1.17 SPIRITUAL ALCHEMY

Since the north-east direction indicates the movement from cool towards warmth it is represented by yin moving to yang ▬▬ . It also indicates a progression towards a balancing of the masculine/feminine, positive/ negative, extroverted/introverted polarities (+ –). Elemental Fire is an influence in both its directional and cyclical activity (+ +). The spirituality of Falcon expresses the masculine emphasis (+). So the combination of these essential factors (+ -, + + +) indicates a largely outgoing personality with some tendency towards introspection.

The strong influence of elemental Fire indicates that Falcons are great generators of activity, and always busying themselves. Such a concentration of fire energies might be discerned by a shaman as a powerful outrushing force seeking to express itself through activity. The essence of such activity might be understood as the desire for self-expression. Part of Falcon's life-purpose is to learn to control the Fire that is within so that the vital energies are readily available rather than of use only in flashes. The need is to sustain as well as to initiate, to serve as well as to lead.

1.18 LIFE-CHALLENGES

In their quest for knowledge fashioned by experience, Falcons must learn to cultivate discernment and moderation so that they are not so easily attracted to everything that sparkles or carried away to excesses by every wind of change.

They are likely to find themselves in situations that provide opportunities to curb their impulsiveness and impatience and provide lessons in the value of practising humility and tolerance towards others.

Falcons need to cultivate moderation, patience, compassion, tolerance and humility. They need to curb any tendencies towards impatience, impulsiveness, restlessness, intolerance and compulsion and coercion.

1.19 PRIMARY FUNCTION AND LIFE-PATH

The primary function of Falcon is to gain knowledge through the experience of initiating action. The purpose is to experience one's own separateness and to discover that while it is possible to function independently without dependence on others, happiness comes through sharing. However, Falcons need to be themselves and not what they think others want them to be, so it is a path to lead them to find themselves and to establish their own individuality but in harmony with others.

On this path they are fired by the enthusiasm to get things started, and motivated by such driving force that they try to push through the problems they encounter head-on rather than pause to consider ways around them.

It is a journey of experience, of daring to be adventurous, and its lessons are the recognition of the importance of completing what one has started and that the safest and less troublesome way to tackle an obstacle in one's path is often to walk around it rather than to try to force it out of the way.

The need to develop spiritual ideals or ethical principles to meet life's challenges will be in evidence.

The capacity to initiate creative ideas and to bring them into practical realization will be a prime function, though many of them may only be short-lived.

There is a suggestion of compassionate leadership exerted like a parent.

The prime purpose might be summarised as the discernment, through experience, of what is of true value and what is false, and the acceptance of personal responsibility.

1.20 THE I CHING TRIGRAM: Ch'ien. Heaven.

This trigram suggests one-ness and individuality. It also represents the creative, conceptual power that is propelled forward and expresses itself in starting things. It implies that what is created in the present will be experienced in the future. Its realization is that what is set in motion now will come to be experienced next. Its message is: 'Know where your actions will lead', for what Falcons set in motion and initiate will set up ripples which will come into their circle of experience later.

When coupled with Fire it indicates success through effort that is undertaken with perseverance and clarity of mind.

1.21 HOW TO COPE WITH FALCONS

Falcons are less concerned with long-term considerations than with what is happening here and now, or what is likely to come about pretty soon. So you'll interest them most with what is immediate.

Be enthusiastic, positive and to-the-point in dealing with Falcons, but don't be offended by any signs of arrogance, or be provoked if Falcon touches a sensitive spot in your mental armoury. Meet Falcon with tact and courtesy.

Falcons are impatient and get bored easily, so lengthy and detailed explanations are not likely to impress them. They want the highlights, and they want them crisp and clear. If they want the small details they'll ask for them.

Beaver

SUMMARY

Birth dates:	20 April – 20 May (23 October – 22 November in the Southern hemisphere).
Earth influence:	The Growing Time.
Influencing wind:	The East Winds. *Totem:* Eagle.
Direction:	East.
Predominant element:	Earth with Fire.
Elemental clan:	Turtle (Earth) Clan. *Function:* to consolidate.
Birth and animal totem:	Beaver.
Plant totem:	Wild Clover.
Mineral totem:	Jasper bloodstone.
Polarity totem:	Snake.
Affinity colour:	Yellow.
Personality:	Determined. Resourceful. Opinionated. Methodical.
Feelings:	Highly strung.
Nature:	Industrious.
Intention:	Possession.
Positive traits:	Strong-willed. Businesslike. Persistent.
Negative traits:	Possessive. Self-indulgent. Inflexible.
Sex-drive:	Demanding.
Compatibilities:	Woodpeckers, Brown Bears and Geese.
Conscious aim:	Security through possession.
Subconscious desire:	Freedom from attachments.
Life-path:	To discover and possess that which has lasting value.
I Ching trigram:	☲ Li. Clinging fire. Success through persistence.
Spiritual alchemy:	Yin predominates.
Must cultivate:	Adaptability. Enterprise. Compassion.
Must avoid:	Possessiveness. Inflexibility. Stubbornness.
Starting totems:	Beaver. Eagle. Turtle. Wild clover. Jasper bloodstone. Snake.

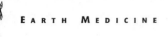

2.Beaver

2.1 BIRTH MONTH: 20 April – 20 May

2.2 EARTH INFLUENCE: The Growing Time

The Growing Time is the second of the spring cycles and marks the period when grasses develop and spread rapidly to transform the landscape. It indicates a period of growth in the natural cycle that involves dramatic change. It is the time of new life putting down roots and securing the stability of Earth.

It is the time when spring is stirring to its fullest expression with trees in full leaf, flowers in bloom, and the creative forces of Nature evident everywhere.

People with birthdays during the Growing Time are the 'earthiest', or most materialistic, of those born during the three spring cycles, and possess an impetus towards growth and expansion in material directions.

This period also includes a crossover point in the season cycle – the East point on the Wheel of the Year – which comes mid-way between the Spring Equinox on 21 March and the Summer Solstice on 21 June. It coincides with the last day of April, but was more often celebrated among northern peoples as May Day. In ancient times among northern cultures, it was a festival of union and initiation, and emphasized the time in life of romance and sexual awareness. It also recognized the period of testing that anyone who searches for the unison of mind, body and spirit must undergo.

People of this time are likely to be romantics and to be sexually aware, and though materialistic by nature they will have an inner desire for the longer-lasting satisfaction that is derived from mental and spiritual things. The totality of their lifetime experiences might be described as initiatory, for they are involved in a transition from one level of their being to another and such experiences can often be traumatic and sometimes painful.

2.3 SOLAR INFLUENCES

This is the month when the spring season reaches its zenith though the solar energies are still waxing towards their peak. So people of this time will express creativity in some form as well as organizational skills. If the solar energies are being expressed negatively there will be displays of extravagance and arrogance.

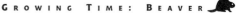

The temperament will be warm and affectionate by nature, but it can be quite chilling and even vengeful to anyone whom they consider to be an adversary. The related Sun sign is Taurus.

2.4 INFLUENCING WIND: The East Winds
DIRECTION: East

The East Winds bring to the Growing Time a similar emphasis on far-sightedness which we encountered the previous month with Awakening Time people. But since the Growing Time is the period of rooting rather than of budding, and of blossoming forth from a stable base, those born at this time will show a greater emphasis on the things they can touch and handle rather than on ideas.

In others words, their far-sightedness is likely to be concerned with the security that is felt from making things last beyond the present and the immediate future. It will be more concerned with the material aspects of life than with the intangibles of mental ideas and spiritual principles.

However, the East is the direction of the dawn and awakening – the time to take steps to turn dreams into practical reality. So the spiritual influence we saw emphasized in the Awakening Time is still there but in the Growing Time it is being directed more to an opening up from within to an expression that is without – like the petals of a blossoming flower. So while Awakening Time people like to start new things, Growing Time people are more inclined to want to stay put to appreciate what is at hand all around them. Whereas Awakening Time people are likely to go forth in exuberance even in the rains of adversity, Growing Time people are inclined to see the world from where they stand, even in a raindrop.

The totem of the East is the *eagle* which is described in section 1.4.

2.5 INFLUENCING ELEMENTS: Earth with Fire

Growing Time people are influenced by the directional power of elemental Fire which imbues them with vibrancy but it is the energy to get things done rather than to do things. Its radiance is in the enthusiasm for the things that attract them and which is also its driving power. Its influence is apparent in their creativity and versatility, and also in their practicability in transforming what they see around them into the things they consider essential for their own security and well-being.

Since Fire is associated with the spirit, one of the great realizations that Growing Time people need to experience is that there are spiritual qualities within the material. In other words, they are being encouraged to see beyond external realities and to attain the far-sightedness of the Eagle to see beyond the reaches of matter.

Elemental Earth influences those born in the Growing Time in its cyclic activity. Its effect is to cause them to want to hold on to material possessions and to be purposeful and determined. Expressed negatively it will make them appear inflexible and resistant to change, and possessive.

The polarity of Fire is + and of Earth –.

2.6 ELEMENTAL CLAN: Turtle Clan

Growing Time people are related to the turtle Clan which is the influence of elemental Earth. It is, perhaps, not difficult to understand why, of all the animals, the turtle was chosen by many Amerindian tribes as a symbolic representation of Earth. It has a hard outer shell which contains a living being. It rises slowly out of the water as land once rose out of the sea, and the shape and firmness of the turtle's back is similar to the appearance of land viewed from the sea. Once the turtle has created its young by laying eggs, it leaves them to fend for themselves, just as Mother Earth does with us.

Since elemental Earth contributed the properties of stability and cohesion to the form and shape of matter, these same characteristics will be in evidence in the personalities of those influenced by this element and born into the Turtle Clan.

People of the Turtle Clan will feel a strong need to establish a stable base from which to operate and to put down roots, and they will want to have solid and constructive things around them.

They will make progress slowly and carefully, primarily through the application of persistence and tenacity. It is the Earth element in their make-up which enables them to make firm progress and to establish solid achievements. However, they need to learn to keep these Earth energies in balance, otherwise stability may become mere stubbornness and inflexibility, which can result in frustration for themselves and for those around them. Firmness can become a hardness of spirit with a subsequent lack of sympathy, understanding and compassion for others, and their natural carefulness can degenerate into clumsiness and inconsideration. Persistence and tenacity, too, are positive qualities but imbalance can turn them into a reluctance to 'let go' to the point where Growing Time people who find themselves in difficult situations allow themselves to become martyrs.

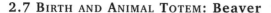

2.7 BIRTH AND ANIMAL TOTEM: Beaver

The birth and animal totem for those born between 20 April and 20 May is the Beaver, an amphibious rodent which can grow to 90–100 cm (3–4 ft) long and weigh over 30 kg (70 lb).

Although a land animal, the beaver's cardiovascular system enables it to store oxygen and to stay underwater for a quarter of an hour or more. Its nimble front paws enable it to hold food and nibble like a hamster, as well as to carry through the water the materials with which to fashion its habitat.

Its hind legs have webbed, paddle-like paws which enable it to move through the water at high speed. It has soft, brown fur which is lubricated and waterproofed with oil from its musk glands. It has a broad, flat, scaly tail which serves as a rudder when the animal is swimming and as a balancer when it is on land.

Beavers are the architects and construction engineers of the animal world, who can transform their environment to provide for their own security and comfort. They are able to cut down trees and branches with their sharp teeth to provide the materials from which to construct dams to create a pond or lake in which they can build their lodges from sticks and mud. They can cut canals which may extend for hundreds of feet and build on different layers with locks to maintain water levels. Beavers use these locks to maintain a deep body of water at a constant level throughout the year.

Like their animal totem, people born in the Growing Time are constant hard workers. Like beavers, they are always busying themselves with making alterations and improvements to their homes and to their working conditions. The purpose of all their activity is security and contentment, both of which are essential qualities for their well-being.

Beaver people are adaptable and creative. They are patient and persevering, too, which means that they can usually end up with having what they had set their hearts and minds on. They have creativity and flair, and consequently are usually good at reconstructing, on emotional as well as material levels.

Quick to learn and nimble with their hands as well as their minds, Beaver people are good at 'engineering' events to suit themselves, even to the point of reorganizing the lives of others around them in order to improve their own living or working environment. The changes they bring about are not entirely selfish, however, but generally benefit others as well as themselves.

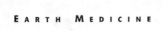

Stability is important to Beaver people, so they look for lasting rather than passing relationships, and they are 'hangers on' to whatever they regard of value.

2.8 PLANT TOTEM: Wild clover

Wild clover (*Trifolium pratense*), sometimes called red clover – a perennial plant that carpets fields and areas of North America and also parts of Europe, was a totem plant among many Indian tribes. It has a short, clinging rootstock which produces a number of hairy stems that grow about 50 cm (20 inches) high. The leaves have three oval-shaped leaflets and it has single flowerheads with reddish or reddish-white flowers.

The plant nourishes the soil with nitrogen, and it provides bees with a rich source of pollen, which makes superb honey. It makes a fine animal fodder.

Clover was used for medicinal purposes by the Indians, and it also figured prominently in European folk medicine. It was used as a remedy for constipation and for a sluggish appetite. The flowering tops of the plant, when made into a tea, were said to stimulate the liver and the gall bladder. Tea made from the leaves was said to calm the nerves when agitated by pressure or stress.

Like their plant totem, whose roots do not go down deep but cling to the earth to provide a lush carpet of vegetation, Beaver people have a down-to-earth attitude and cling to the feeling of stability that earthy things give. And as the plant feeds the soil and animals with its nutrients so Beaver people provide support and sustenance for the people and projects they are associated with. The clover nectar provides bees with the means to make superb honey, and Beaver people, too, are able to sweeten and nourish the lives of others as well as attaining contentment for themselves.

2.9 MINERAL TOTEM: Jasper bloodstone

Jasper is a dull cryptocrystalline quartz which comes in reddish brown, brown, yellow and green colorations. The jasper associated with people of the Growing Time is the green variety that is flecked with reddish spots and is known as bloodstone or heliotrope. Heliotrope means 'sun-reflecting' and, significantly, as green is the colour of plants that reach upwards towards the Sun, so heliotrope was seen as an aid to uplifting the human consciousness towards the spiritual Sun, and so was considered as a tool of the spirit. The bloodstone was thus highly regarded among all

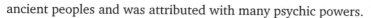

ancient peoples and was attributed with many psychic powers.

The red flecks contain iron and help the stone to act as a styptic which stems bleeding. Amerindians used the stone as a protection against wounds and insect bites and to stem the flow of blood from nose-bleeds or cuts. It was also used to heal stomach aches and intestinal disorders by being worn in the navel.

It was used to stimulate the power centres of the Energic Body (the chakras) by being moved up the spine in circular motions. Its slow subtle vibrations were thought to be transmitted to the chakras and helped to align their energy patterns. Indeed, it was as an 'aligner' – as a 'bringer of things into line' so that they worked in effective relationship with one another – that the bloodstone was most regarded.

The bloodstone was also used to prepare a tonic. It was put in a container of water for a day or two and left in the sunlight. When the stone was removed, the water was consumed. It was thought that the water absorbed energies from the stone, and its effect as a general tonic was to help to balance the body's subtle energies.

Like their totem stone, Beaver people also have an intrinsic ability to bring harmony into the lives of others when their energies are used in an outgoing way. But when these powers, whether intentionally or subconsciously, are directed to entirely selfish purposes or to manipulate others for personal gain, they are likely to have the opposite effect and to stir up confusion, contention, and even pain.

2.10 POLARITY TOTEM: Snake

European myths about the snake, and especially some religious allegories, have turned it into a creature that many find repulsive and fearful. But among aboriginal cultures, the snake was highly regarded, not least because of its great transforming powers as it frequently shed its skin. Among Amerindians, the snake was respected as 'a teacher of wisdom'.

Beaver people have the urge to make things permanent on the physical plane, and the ability to convert ideas into form. They also want to acquire and possess. What Beavers can learn from the complementary Snake is the desirability of eliminating what is not essential to spiritual progress and to material well-being.

Snake can teach Beaver that material possessions alone can offer little lasting satisfaction, and that it is sharing them, not having them, that brings fulfilment: the greatest pleasures of life are those that are shared.

Then the attitude is transformed from one of 'That's mine' to 'That's ours'. Beavers will make more of their personality assets when they have acquired some of Snake's concern with probing the mysteries of life and discovered some of the deeper realities behind all outward appearances.

2.11 PERSONALITY EXPRESSION
Adult

Practical, reliable and methodical. Beaver people are sticklers and will generally persevere until they achieve their objective.

They are home-loving, and value their personal comfort sometimes to the point of opulence. They require a peaceful and harmonious atmosphere around them, otherwise they are likely to become nervous, irritable and highly strung, and prone to possible digestive troubles.

The Beaver person is endowed with practical aptitudes and with a certain manual dexterity, but there is also a sharp artistic and aesthetic sense which shows itself in refined visual 'taste'. Beavers are attracted by the beauty of things, whether it is a tree in blossom, a flower in bloom, or the artistry and craftsmanship displayed in a work of art, or elegant clothes. For their world is the world of physical sensations.

Beaver people are conservative and cautious in their attitudes, and since they often only believe in what they see with their own eyes, are generally orthodox in any religious or philosophical thinking.

The male is usually steady, capable and productive, with a clear sense of purpose. Since security is so fundamental to him, his ambitions are unlikely to include taking risks.

The female has a keen dress sense, and though her practicability will incline her towards comfortable clothes, she has a flair for pretty things. She likes a warm and cosy atmosphere, so she is usually a good home-maker.

Positive traits: Practical. Reliable. Patient. Businesslike. Persistent. Determined. Strong-willed. Affectionate.

Negative traits: Possessive. Lazy. Self-indulgent. Inflexible. Stubborn. Resentful.

Vocational possibilities: Agriculture. Business and commerce. Cooking. Entertaining. Housekeeping. Investing. Mining. Music. Military. Property. Natural sciences. Theatre. Sculpting. Writing.

Child

The Beaver infant is likely to present two main problems – its possessive-ness and its stubbornness. Infant Beaver doesn't like sharing. If another child picks up its toy, infant Beaver will bawl its head off. Infant Beaver needs to be weaned off its possessiveness, but it must be done with gentleness and assurance.

At school the young Beaver is likely to be more of a plodder than a high-flyer, but the Beaver child has good powers of concentration, so its progress should be steady and sure. Young Beavers respond well to sound discipline and clear, no-nonsense rules which provide them with the security of knowing where they stand. They are usually the more mature members of their peer group.

Parent

The male Beaver finds delight in parenthood and is usually happy to devote time to his children, responding to their needs with warmth and affection. Since he tends to put much emphasis on material things, he runs the risk of spoiling his children with too many 'goodies', particularly his daughters. He is likely to set a high standard for his children, but he is con-siderate, tolerant and understanding when they are very young, but usually more demanding as they get older.

The Beaver mother is adoring and devoted to her young offspring, but as they grow older she is likely to become more demanding and will not tolerate laziness or untidiness.

As the children develop into teenagers, the Beaver parent tends to find some difficulty in bridging the generation gap and understanding the ideas and attitudes of teenage offspring which seem to be so very different from their own. The fault, of course, lies in their own conservatism and rigidity.

2.12 ROMANCE AND SEX

Beavers can be sensual and exciting lovers with a keen sexual appetite that can be quite demanding and even lustful. Their love-making is slow and deliberate.

They are loyal and devoted lovers, but their need to feel safe and secure causes them to seek constant assurance that their partner feels equally for them too. Should their partner give cause for them to be suspicious or arouse their jealousy, they are likely to blow their top and become overbearing, requiring constant proof of their partner's loyalty. Emotionally, a stable and loving relationship is absolutely essential to them.

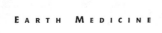

The Beaver male can be a real charmer, bringing all the romantic little touches into the relationship. His sexual appetite is as insatiable as his stomach.

The female Beaver likes her man to be masculine and aggressive without being domineering for she hates being ordered about and told what to do. She just likes her man to be manly.

Compatibilities: Beavers are compatible with Woodpeckers, Brown Bears and Geese (those born between 21 June and 21 July, 22 August and 21 September, and 22 December and 19 January).

Spiritual sexuality: (–) The basic spiritual sexuality of Beavers is feminine, but this has nothing to do with gender. It means that Beavers are usually receptive and introverted in their attitudes and desires, and are responsive rather than aggressive. In physical relationships it means they are more likely to respond to the initiative of their partner rather than taking the initiative themselves.

2.13 Health

In general Beaver people have a robust constitution, but through their liking for food and the good things of life, and a tendency towards self-indulgence, they may become prone to heart conditions and kidney troubles later in life.

Their most vulnerable area is the throat. They are susceptible to throat infections and suffer from sore throats more frequently than most people. The other area most prone to health problems is the uterus or prostrate gland and the bladder.

2.14 Affinity Colour: Yellow

Yellow is an inspiring and expressive colour, for it is the ray of the imagination and of fantasy. It expands the mind and stimulates the mental faculties. It is the colour of spontaneity and of the yearning for variety. So Growing Time people will be stimulated by change and variety. They will be imaginative, but with a tendency to fantasize.

Yellow is associated with the intellect and indicates a capacity to understand. What is that Beaver people are seeking to understand? Primarily – though they may not be aware of this – it is seeking to understand themselves, though there is also a need to make sense of the world around them.

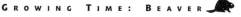

2.15 ADVANTAGEOUS TIMES

Best months of the year for Beaver people are from 20 April to 20 May, 22 September to 22 October, and 22 December to 19 January.

Best day of the week is Friday.

Best times of the day are from 5 a.m. to 7 a.m. and 5 p.m. to 7 p.m.

2.16 OUTWARD (CONSCIOUS) AIM AND
INNER (SUBCONSCIOUS) DESIRE

The driving force of Beaver people is towards the security that comes through *having*. Their urge is towards possessions, and to obtain the satisfaction that possession gives. Their aim is to consolidate and to make secure.

But the desire of Beaver's unconscious self is to find liberation, which is freedom from attachments. It means not being possessed by possessions or obsessed with them. So Beavers are likely to be drawn into situations where they are being led to find a link between the material and the spiritual.

It is the link which is their 'pearl of great price', for a purpose of their life is to rise above the fascination of the senses and to discover that the contentment they crave lies above attachment to merely physical things.

2.17 SPIRITUAL ALCHEMY

As we have seen, Beaver people are affected by a combination of the 'directional' influence of elemental Fire (+) and the cyclical activity of elemental Earth (−). Elemental Earth activates the need to establish secure foundations and to amass. But just as the Earth itself could not exist as a living entity without the Fire that is at its core, as well as the light and warmth that comes from the Fire of the Sun, so Beaver people need to tap into an inner power to motivate them as well as the outer light to enable them to see where they are going.

What is being implied here is that clarity of vision is needed to put a firm foundation under anything that is being done to accomplish one's purpose. Without that vision, whatever is attained has no lasting value for it, too, will be affected by the immutable Law of Change. The firm foundation Beavers truly need is of spiritual values. This, for all their busyness and honest endeavour, is often overlooked by industrious Beaver.

The directional influence is one of the receptive changing to the active (− +) and the spiritual emphasis of the Beaver is feminine (−). So the combination of these polarities (+ −, − + and −) indicates a busy, active personality that wants to be seen doing and acquiring things, being pulled by a strong balancing factor towards receptivity and assimilation. When under pressure, therefore, or suffering stress, the impulse to thrust one's way through by further activity needs to be resisted for the spiritual metabolism is best left to work quietly to find inner ways to align to change and to bring the individual into equilibrium.

2.18 LIFE-CHALLENGES

Though Beaver people have a strong feeling about the need to have security and solidity of physical things around them, they are learning in this lifetime to tread the material path without becoming too rooted in earthly things and forming such attachment to them that they become dependent on them. It is this attachment and dependency, taken almost to the point of addiction, that causes them pain and suffering.

Indeed, it is when this tendency to become enmeshed in attachments is extended into personal relationships to the point where it becomes possessiveness, that they undergo their worst emotional traumas.

Beavers need to cultivate flexibility and adaptability and to overcome those tendencies towards rigidity, frigidity and over-indulgence of the sensual appetites.

2.19 PRIMARY FUNCTION AND LIFE-PATH

The primary function of Beaver is to build solid and secure foundations that are lasting. That final word when considered alongside the link that Beaver has with the polar opposite, Snake, provides a clue to the inner path of the soul. Beavers busy themselves with seeking material ownership as proof of their value, but these are only shadows of what they inwardly strive to discover and to build upon, which are the things that have eternal value. Beavers desire freedom, but true liberation comes only when the things that they have are no longer attachments.

There is an inherent capacity to work creatively within limitations and this develops an ability to manage material things.

Beaver's life-path leads to the discovery of ways to soothe inner wounds that cause suffering in everyday life, and to learning to bring compassionate understanding to others in pain.

The prime purpose might be summarized as: to manifest and to manage.

2.20 THE I CHING TRIGRAM: Li. Clinging Fire.

Bright, clear and logical. Expresses itself in pleasure, satisfaction, sensuality and persistence.

When coupled with Earth it suggests the need to be externally flexible so that the inner nature can retain its steadfastness in times of difficulty. It implies success through perseverance.

2.21 HOW TO COPE WITH BEAVERS

Be a good listener. Beavers like handing out advice and expressing their own thoughtful points of view. Beavers are gregarious, and they won't thank you for trying to out-talk them.

Compliment them on what they have recently acquired or achieved. If you're invited into their home you will find plenty there worthy of your appreciation.

Beavers thrive on praise and appreciation. Indeed, they almost glow from the warmth it brings them. But don't try flattery. Beavers hate imitations and anything that is not genuine or smacks of falsehood or trickery. Be sincere about the nice things you say.

Be careful about offering advice. Beavers often regard uninvited advice as interference, especially when it concerns their private and domestic life. Beavers are rarely so proud that they are reluctant to seek advice, especially from those they trust and respect.

Deer

SUMMARY

Birth dates:	21 May – 20 June (23 November to 21 December in the Southern hemisphere).
Earth influence:	The Flowering Time.
Influencing wind:	The East Winds. *Totem:* Eagle.
Direction:	South-east.
Predominant elements:	Air with Fire.
Elemental clan:	Butterfly (Air) Clan.
Birth and animal totem:	Deer.
Plant totem:	Mullein.
Mineral totem:	Agate.
Polarity totem:	Owl.
Affinity colour:	Orange.
Personality:	Quick. Alert. Talkative. Congenial. Moody.
Feelings:	Sensitive but superficial.
Intention:	Versatility.
Nature:	Lively.
Positive traits:	Friendly. Witty. Intellectual.
Negative traits:	Inconsistent. Restless. Lazy. Despondent.
Sex-drive:	Titillating.
Compatibilities:	Crows and Otters.
Conscious aim:	To bring together.
Subconscious desire:	Mastery of the mind.
Life-path:	Co-ordination.
I Ching trigram:	⚌ Tui. The Joyful Lake. Success comes through endurance.
Spiritual alchemy:	Yang predominates.
Must cultivate:	Concentration. Persistence. Sympathy.
Must avoid:	Moodiness. Inconsistency. Superficiality.
Starting totems:	Deer. Eagle. Butterfly. Mullein. Agate. Owl.

3. Deer

3.1 BIRTH MONTH: 21 May – 20 June

3.2 EARTH INFLUENCE: The Flowering Time

The Flowering Time is the last cycle of the spring season and is the time when the seeds that were planted in the soil have germinated and are now taking the eventual shape of the fully grown plants.

It compares with the times of youth when the individual is growing into a 'fully grown' human being. It is the time of a great influx of knowledge, but when true understanding is often blocked by the headstrong exuberance of youth.

It is a time of expanding awareness when the world around is seen from a wider perspective. So people born between 21 May and 20 June in the Flowering Time have a capacity to come into a fuller realization of their own inherent potential and their own personal role in the overall scheme of things, though to do so they must apply the extended vision that is available to them and stretch their senses. It means taking opportunities to exercise their intuition in order to comprehend the things that are beyond the range of near-to-the-ground physical senses.

The Flowering Time is the period of transition from spring to summer when the trees are in full leaf and the flowers are blossoming and the whole of Nature is at the height of her creative brilliance.

3.3 SOLAR INFLUENCES

This is the month when the solar energies are waxing to their peak at the Summer Solstice. People born at this time express their creativity intensely and rapidly, usually through some means of bringing attention to themselves. They will be active and versatile though prone to a moodiness that can be as stifling as the atmosphere under a heavy cloud on a sultry summer's day.

They have a warm temperament and an affectionate nature but when out of sorts they can be extremely trying to those closest to them.

The related sign in Sun astrology is Gemini.

3.4 INFLUENCING WIND: East Winds
DIRECTION: South-east

The miraculous energizing power that bursts into new life with the arrival of spring reaches its peak with this third Time of the season when the emphasis moves from awakening and activating to that of transformation. The influence of the East Winds during the Flowering Time can be likened to the period of youth which is a period of undergoing experiences for the first time. The East Winds bring the quality of fearlessness, which is a quality of youth, who rarely contemplate the dangers inherent in a situation before taking action.

As with people of the two earlier spring cycles, Flowering Time people will have a need for far-sightedness, openness, and enlightenment important to their self-development, but there will be a greater urge towards change and the stimulation that comes from moving from one situation to another.

They will reflect something of the spirit of transformation which causes trees and plants to blossom and changes the environment by its touch. It is that vital essence that *changes* things.

The totem of the East is the *eagle*, which is described under the Awakening Time (Falcon). See Section 1.4.

3.5 INFLUENCING ELEMENTS: **Air with Fire**

The power of elemental Fire, which is associated with the East, provides those born in the Flowering Time with an inner urge to want to change what comes within their reach. What they often fail to recognize is that the Fire comes from within themselves and the most important change of all to make is to oneself.

People born in the Flowering Time are usually bright and sparkling personalities with an abundance of energy for the things that attract them, but are less motivated, and even lethargic about the concerns of companions and colleagues. They even blow hot and cold over some of their own interests, to the consternation of those closest to them.

They are also strongly influenced by elemental Air, which is associated with the mind and with thoughts and ideas and with change and movement.

3.6 ELEMENTAL CLAN: **Butterfly Clan (Air)**

Flowering Time people are born into the Butterfly Clan, a clan ruled by elemental Air. The butterfly is a good representation of Air because it is always on the move, constantly shifting its position from one place to another, often unexpectedly.

People born between 21 May and 20 June are like the butterfly – flitting from one flower to another in search of nectar but staying only for a short time before fluttering off to another source. It is as if they are driven by some insatiable curiosity which leads them on a constant journey of exploration, seeking here and searching there, fascinated by what comes into their view but rarely enough for them to stay with it.

Just as butterflies help the plants to pollinate, so Flowering Time people help others with the new ideas and fresh energy they bring.

3.7 BIRTH AND ANIMAL TOTEM: Deer

The swift-moving deer is the birth and animal totem for those born in the Flowering Time.

Although there are many different species of deer, ranging widely in size and weight, they have one thing in common – their gracefulness. The stags have antlers that start to grow in early summer and are fully grown by the mating season in late autumn. They shed the antlers each year around January and February before the young are born in the spring, and it is when they are without antlers that the stags are at their most vulnerable.

Stags and does live in separate groups until the mating season arrives. Then the stags compete with one another for a mate, though they rarely fight to the death. After mating they live in small herds for a while.

Deer blend well with the environment, and are sensitive to every sound and movement. They emit a number of different sounds, but the most common is a bleat like that of a sheep, through it can be a shrieking sound if the animal is frightened or in danger. Deer feed on vegetation – mostly grass, heather, the shoots of plants, and the bark of trees. Twins, and even triplets, are commonly born to the does.

Like their animal totem, Deer people are sensitive, alert and fast-moving. They are intuitive and can readily sense the feelings of others. Since their own feelings and emotions are fast-moving, they are likely to have experienced the moods that other people might find themselves more deeply immersed in. Deer people therefore can be compassionate and understanding.

Deer people do listen but not always attentively. Their thoughts race so quickly that what they hear often starts off a train of thought within their own mind and stirs up their emotions so they feel they have to express these immediately. As a result they have what to some is an annoying tendency to interrupt a conversation and not allow the person who is talking to finish what they are trying to say.

Deer people like beauty and beautiful things – and beautiful people too. Just watch a young male Deer when a beautiful girl comes within range! But it is not always surface beauty that attracts them. They have the discernment to recognize the beauty that lies beneath the skin.

They have a resourcefulness that makes it possible for them to make something attractive out of simple, basic materials. This need to create beauty expresses itself not only physically but emotionally too, and they are able to draw the best out of the people around them.

Like their animal totem, Deer people like the company of members of their own sex and have a willingness to share what they have in common. Such relationships often outlast those with the opposite sex, where they may find difficulty in settling into a single, permanent relationship.

As the deer bounds from one place to another, so Deer people frequently leap from one idea or situation to another, and through not staying with one thing long enough they often fail to accomplish what they set out to do. They have a wild, uncontrollable side to their nature which makes it difficult sometimes for others to understand them, and, indeed, for them to understand themselves. Part of the purpose of their life is to learn the value of discipline, consistency and persistence.

Deer people have difficulty in evaluating time and the expenditure of energy, with the consequence that their lives are not organized in the most effective way.

3.8 PLANT TOTEM: Mullein

Mullein(*Verbascum thapsus*) is a plant with thick, velvety leaves, and densely packed flower spikes. It grows up to 180 cm (6 ft) tall and is found on wasteland and wild places and in fields. It is sometimes called the flannel plant or fluffweed. It is also known as Aaron's rod. This is because its stems have a staff-like appearance and the leaves have tiny hairs which give the appearance of a white coating and flannel-like appearance.

The yellow, five-petalled flowers grow on tall flower spikes close to the stem. They are in bloom from July to August.

Mullein was regarded as a versatile and helpful plant with many soothing qualities. It was used among Amerindians to treat chest ailments and coughs, and also for intestinal disorders. Its leaves were used in a poultice to treat wounds and sores.

As a tea, mullein was said to be beneficial to the kidneys and the bladder. The oil from crushed, fresh mullein flowers was used to remove warts.

Dried mullein leaves were used by some American Indians in a smoking mixture to relieve asthma and lung congestion.

Like their plant totem, Deer people are generally versatile and helpful, with a tendency to rise up above most others in their endeavours or to be noticeable in their activities, although they have a woolly side to their nature.

3.9 MINERAL TOTEM: Agate

Agate is chalcedony, a waxy form of quartz which often lines cavities in rocks and has a banded appearance. These irregularities are caused by differences in decomposition. Its colours vary from white to grey, from blue to green, and brown and black. Agate's emphasis is on material need and this is why it became associated by Westerners with good luck.

A variety of agate is onyx, which has stripes of black and white or brown and white, or green. Onyx was sometimes called the 'listening' stone because it was said to aid meditation and help its user to 'listen' to the inner voice of the conscience or High Self.

Deer people should wear agate as a pendant or necklace or ring since it has a stabilizing effect on the subtle energies of the aura if worn next to the skin. It also helps the chakras in the solar plexus, heart and throat areas to work together in harmony. It is a help, too, in stabilizing emotions, and this is important for Deer people who can suffer the effects of their emotions running wild.

Deer people are generally so quick to move from one idea or situation to another that they don't stay with it long enough to recognize the truth that lies within it. Their mineral totem can be a great help in stabilizing their energies so they can overcome this difficulty.

Agate was regarded as a healing stone among many Amerindian tribes.

3.10 POLARITY TOTEM: Owl

Deer people need the guidance of Owl, their polar opposite, in order to train and widen the intellect so that it can become the tool for extending their awareness beyond what is obvious in the immediate environment.

Deer loves to amass information, but does not co-ordinate it well enough to put it to the most effective use. Owl is a visionary, the wise old bird who can help Deer to control the intellect and to reach out into the regions of intuitive knowledge and thereby to see beyond what is immediate.

3.11 PERSONALITY EXPRESSION
Adult

Congenial, adaptable, bubbly and expressive, Deer people thrive on a variety of change. They have a lively sensitivity but their oscillation between confidence and discouragement, high spirits and depression, can give an impression that they are two distinct personalities.

They can be charming, engaging, and full of fun, but also irritable and sarcastic and dampeners.

Deer people crave variety and are continually searching for exciting diversion. They have the mental and manual dexterity to handle a wide variety of tasks, often with considerable skill, but get easily bored with one particular activity and often lack the commitment and practicability to make a real success of it. They loathe drudgery and monotony and routine.

They are good communicators, and can talk about almost anything to almost anybody. Possibly they talk too much and listen too little to get the most out of a relationship. They absorb information readily, though they rarely stay with it long enough to know it thoroughly, and are prone to making snap judgements before they know all the essential facts.

Deer people require plenty of mental activity or they become easily bored. Indeed, they live in a world of ideas and thrive on mental challenge, frequently taking on more than they can manage with the result that they become prone to nervous exhaustion.

They'll change their job almost as easily as changing their clothes. Indeed, they are natural moonlighters and likely to be supplementing their income from one job with what they can make from a sideline or two.

Punctuality is not one of their strong points and it is not always because of lack of organization. It sometimes just seems to happen that way.

Positive traits: Adaptable. Versatile. Intellectual. Witty. Logical. Talkative. Lively.

Negative traits: Moody. Changeable. Restless. Cunning. Inconsistent. Superficial. Lazy.

Vocational possibilities: Aviation. Communications. Dancing. Electrical engineering. Electronics. Linguistics. Motor industry. Media. Office work. Politics. Public relations. Sports. Writing.

Child

Deer infants are bundles of energy – quick, alert, lively and into everything. As they develop into children, it becomes evident that they have an active imagination and can become so engrossed in the world of make-believe that they run the risk of carrying it with them into their teens and right into adulthood, confusing illusion with reality. It is not a question of telling lies, nor of imagining things. The Deer will be convinced that the fantasy really happened.

Deer children need to be encouraged to express themselves and to be given a sense of direction as they may lack the patience and concentration to learn a subject thoroughly. Their quick minds are all too often satisfied in just skimming the surface of a subject.

Parent

Deer make devoted, even doting parents, and can be so carried away by their enthusiasm to provide their offspring with the best of everything that they will make almost any sacrifice to provide it. The rub comes later in life when they then expect their children to respond with the same kind of devotion and are likely to suffer bitter disappointment.

3.12 ROMANCE AND SEX

It is easy to interpret Deer's natural friendliness as blatant flirtatiousness. Deer males are expert at chatting up women. Their fascinating conversation can have a woman believing almost everything they say, and their manner can be captivating enough to charm her into submission. Deer females are engaging conversationalists too. At their best they are quick-witted, amusing and alluring. At their worst – well, there's just no stopping them.

Both male and female Deer like titillation before sexual involvement and will follow this through with a performance that is almost as athletic as their vocal and mental agility. And they tend to talk even during their love-making. Since versatility is a key to the Deer temperament, fidelity is not usually one of their strong points.

The way to the heart of a Deer person is to share their interests. But for their part, they shy away from sharing in domestic chores, and though they enjoy food, cooking is rarely among their enthusiasms.

Compatibilities: Deer are compatible with Crows and Otters (those born between 22 September and 22 October, and between 20 January and 18 February).

Spiritual sexuality: (+). The basic spiritual sexuality of Deer is masculine, which means that Deer people are usually extroverted and active in their attitudes and desires. They are likely to take the initiative in sexual activity.

3.13 HEALTH

People born in the Flowering Time have such active minds that they tend to stay up late and seldom get enough sleep. As they are prone to live on their nerves, nervous exhaustion is a constant threat to their well-being.

The Flowering Time is related to the arms and the shoulders of the external body and these areas are prone to health problems. The internal organs most vulnerable are the lungs and bronchial passages, so care must be taken that colds and influenza do not develop into bronchitis and pneumonia.

Other health problems are likely to have their root in the liver and to toxics in the system.

3.14 AFFINITY COLOUR: Orange

As orange lies between the yellow and the red rays, and yellow is associated with the mental and red with the physical, orange is regarded as a bridge between the mental and the physical. It brings the power of the mind (yellow) into physical activity (red). The influence of orange, therefore, is to energize thought – to bring creativity into manifestation. Learning to do just that is part of the life-purpose of Deers.

Orange is warm and cheerful, and Deer people are comfortable in a warm and cheerful atmosphere. They respond to an inharmonious atmosphere by curling up within themselves and becoming withdrawn.

3.15 ADVANTAGEOUS TIMES

Best months of the year for Deer people are from 21 May to 20 June, 22 August to 22 October and 20 January to 18 February.
Best day of the week is Wednesday.
Best times of the day are from 7 a.m. to 9 a.m. and 7 p.m. to 9 p.m.

3.16 OUTWARD (CONSCIOUS) AIM AND
INNER (SUBCONSCIOUS) DESIRE

The conscious aim of Deer is to link together and to correlate. It is to establish relationships and bring together.

Deer people need to unite their talents and energies rather than separate them. For instance the problem is how to unite the creativity of the mind with the dexterity for manual skills, or how to adapt ideas to the sensory world.

The thought processes of Deer people usually follow the route of logic. But life-experiences will lead them to the need to extend their mental processes beyond the intellect so that they might become masters of the mind rather than servants of it. That is the true intent of their subconscious desire.

3.17 SPIRITUAL ALCHEMY

Deer people are carried on the wind of ideas, from one attractive activity to the next, and with whatever stimulates the mind. They are also driven by an inner Fire that urges them towards changing things. What is needed to balance their energies is to transform their thoughts and ideas into solid and practical reality, and the means to do that are within themselves. They will develop a deeper perspective by staying with a thing long enough to look beneath surface appearances.

The directional influence is of the passive (–) changing to the active (+), and the elemental polarities of Fire is (+) and of Air is also (+). The spiritual sexuality is also masculine. The combination is (– +, + + and +).

3.18 LIFE-CHALLENGES

Deer people are likely to encounter occasional experiences that tend to slow them down. There will seem to be setbacks and circumstances that appear to be binding or restricting. The purpose of such traumas is to slow Deer people down because they are bounding ahead of themselves. They should look upon such limiting situations as blessings in disguise, for they provide opportunities to pause awhile and consider consequences and examine choices. They are a man of 'catching up' with oneself, establishing one's bearings, and facing up to the issues that are of real importance.

Deer people need to develop their powers of concentration and to acquire stability and staying power. They need to avoid restlessness and dissipating their energies in fruitless pursuits, and also to curb their broodiness and ingratitude.

3.19 PRIMARY FUNCTION AND LIFE-PATH

The primary function of Deer people is to co-ordinate that which appears to be contradictory in their lives into a balanced harmony. Their life-path is leading them to a recognition that to find equilibrium they need to bring the intellect and the intuitive faculties, reason and emotion, conscious and subconscious, into balance. Their purpose is to heal the divisions they find within themselves.

Deer people are endowed with a strong sense of curiosity which seems to draw them along a path of new experiences and constant variety. The spiritual purpose of curiosity is the attainment of knowledge, and knowledge, to be of true value, must be applied.

Realization comes to Deer people with the recognition that the knowledge they obtain through experiences must be applied in determining choices. Fulfilment comes to Deer people when that which is of true value is preferred to the irrelevant and transient, and when they stay long enough to gather its fruits.

3.20 The I Ching Trigram: Tui. The Joyous Lake.

This indicates the joy that comes from something well done. It is the joy of satisfaction, and of pleasure in achievement. It represents, too, the desire for contentment – and contentment is a strong need for Deer people, though an elusive one. It stresses, too, that endurance brings success.

3.21 How to Cope with Deer

Don't underestimate Deer's intelligence, so reason with them over difficult issues, but bear in mind their emotional vulnerability. Don't get too intense or emotional.

Be a good listener. Deer like to talk, but they hate being talked down themselves. To the Deer, a good conversationalist is someone who listens to what they have to say.

Deer like variety and hate routine. So look for different ways of presenting them with the ordinary.

Deer are highly strung, so make them feel relaxed and comfortable in your company.

Woodpecker

SUMMARY

Birth dates:	21 June – 21 July (22 December – 19 January in the Southern hemisphere).
Earth influence:	The Long Days Time.
Influencing wind:	South Winds. *Totem:* Mouse.
Direction:	South-south-east.
Predominant element:	Water.
Elemental clan:	Frog (Water) Clan. *Function:* to merge.
Birth and animal totem:	Woodpecker
Plant totem:	Wild rose.
Mineral totem:	Rose quartz.
Polarity totem:	Goose.
Affinity colour:	Rose.
Personality:	Emotional. Sensitive. Protective. Vulnerable.
Feelings:	Maternal/Paternal. Romantic.
Intention:	Devotion.
Nature:	Exacting.
Positive traits:	Imaginative. Tender. Thrifty. Sympathetic.
Negative traits:	Possessive. Moody. Unforgiving.
Sex-drive:	Needful.
Compatibilities:	Snakes, Wolves and Beavers.
Conscious aim:	Emotional unfoldment.
Subconscious desire:	Timeliness.
Life-path:	Assimilation.
I Ching trigram:	☱ Tui. Lake. Desire for contentment.
Spiritual alchemy:	Yin predominates.
Must cultivate:	Intuitiveness. Resourcefulness. Forgiveness.
Must avoid:	Self-pity. Envy. Possessiveness.
Starting totems:	Woodpecker. Mouse. Frog. Wild rose. Rose quartz. Goose.

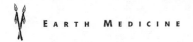
4. Woodpecker

4.1 BIRTH MONTH: 21 June – 21 July

4.2 EARTH INFLUENCE: The Long Days Time

The Long Days Time is the first of the three cycles of the summer season and begins at the Summer Solstice when Nature starts to slow its pace and to grow towards the maturity of bearing fruit. The Long Days Time heralds the fulfilment of the promise of the spring season, which is the abundance that results from a firm rooting in the Earth.

The Summer Solstice, which marks the beginning of the Long Days Time, is the very height of the year when the days are longest and the nights the shortest. It is a time of delight in the great outdoors; a time when the rich, green vegetation is lush and comforting beneath the feet, and when the air is filled with the intoxicating fragrance of flowers.

It can be compared with the time in life when youth reaches adulthood and the period of testing and maturing. People whose birthdays are in the Long Days Time have the potential for bearing much fruit and to grow into the maturity which comes from gaining wisdom through experience and responsibility.

The Long Days Time can also be compared with midday when the Sun reaches its zenith and gives its brightest light and maximum warmth. For people born in this time, a lifetime of testing and developing to bring to maximum potential the inherent qualities they brought with them at birth is indicated.

It is a time, too, of hope and expectation for the long, hot days of summer that still lie ahead, and for the reward of all one's efforts.

So it was that in ancient times the Summer Solstice was the Festival of Expectation.

4.3 SOLAR INFLUENCES

Nature is busy nurturing and protecting all that has been born as the Sun moves to its zenith to herald in the splendour of summer and the joy of alive-ness that the radiance of the Sun brings and which becomes evident everywhere.

Woodpeckers will share the nurturing and protective instincts and the sensitivities that abound in Nature now.

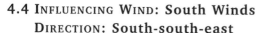

4.4 INFLUENCING WIND: South Winds
DIRECTION: South-south-east

As the rays of the Sun on a bright summer's day are not obscured by clouds but are able to impart warmth and energy to all they touch, so people born in the Long Days Time are brought into incarnation on the warm Winds of the South and influenced by an essence which enables them to develop through the experience of direct contact. The influence of the South Winds is one that enables things to be comprehended 'close to' and to be seen in their true light.

People born in the Long Days Time are influenced by the directional power of the South whose 'maturing' energies operate in a spirit of trust and innocence. Indeed, South is sometimes described as 'the place of Trust and Innocence'.

Let me try to explain that. According to the Amerindian all growing things 'trust' that their early growth has brought enough substance from the Earth to enable them to develop and mature in accordance with the purpose contained within the seed and, of course, to perpetuate themselves. Some might define that as a 'divine' trust that is inherent in growing things themselves.

Applied to the human condition, it means a childlike (but not childish!) dependence on one's own inherent instincts, or that 'inner voice', in finding and fulfilling the purpose of one's life, and not to be sidetracked by the cynicism, illusory fears, false values and guilt complexes of 'adulthood'.

Innocence, to the Indian, does not mean naivity. It means impartiality and objectivity as compared with subjective opinion. It is a state of non-attachment. It is a condition of mind of the higher nature which is not selfish and possessive and sees not the *differences* but the *unity* of the whole and the harmony that is implicit in the duality of male and female and of all life.

Innocence is a state of mind that is required for purity of vision that is included by personal and selfish considerations. It is the awareness of the one-ness that exists between the one who is seeing and with what is seen.

Innocence, to the Indian, means retaining the simplicity of childhood while enjoying the *experience* of living, and being ever-ready to learn from every fresh 'adventure' in being alive so that life itself can continue to be one of excitement, enjoyment and fulfilment.

The power of the South was seen as providing the opportunity to rid oneself of the encumbrances that can obscure the source of those inherent instincts, the 'inner voice', conscience, or whatever name we give to it – the True Self – so that it might be recognized.

The animal associated with the power of the South as a totem by some tribes was not, as one might suppose from the philosophical outline I have given, large and powerful. It was, indeed, one of the smallest and most insignificant – the tiny *mouse*!

The mouse may appear to be completely inappropriate as a totem and a source of teaching. But bear in mind that the Indian considered that every creature had something of value to impart, so do not dismiss the little mouse.

The mouse, in fact, personified the characteristic of comprehending things by getting close to them – by feeling and by touch – because its whiskers were a special organ of touch which enabled it to be sensitive to its immediate surroundings.

The mouse thus perceives things through its *closeness* to them and by its *feelings* towards them. And it is this that is a principal characteristic of the South.

People born in the Long Days Time will be particularly affected by their feelings of closeness and by the closeness of their feelings. The way they act and the decisions they make will be largely determined by their emotions.

4.5 Influencing Elements: Water

Those born in the Long Days Time are influenced by the element associated with the South – elemental Water. An elemental substance indicates how the cosmic forces or spiritual energies being absorbed into the human auric field are primarily *expressed*. Elemental Water which, since ancient times, has been likened to the emotions, finds expression in the feelings. So those born during the Long Days Time will be deeply affected by their emotions and feel things deeply.

Like physical water elemental Water has the quality of fluidity and will flow in whatever direction it is channelled. Emotions, too, have a 'flowing' quality, but if bottled up can be the cause of frustration and bitterness, and even the root cause of some physical illnesses.

As water renews and refreshes, so elemental Water, too, has great transforming qualities. The polarity of Water is receptive (–).

4.6 Elemental Clan: The Frog Clan (Water)

Long Days Time people are born into the Frog Clan and they have an affinity with water. This affinity can have many beneficial effects. For instance, a stroll by the sea or beside a lake or river, or even within hearing of running water, will have a calming effect and help the flow of inspirational and creative thought within them. In times of turmoil or stress, being near water will help to restore their equilibrium and is recommended, too, when it is necessary for them to make vital and important decisions.

As water dissolves and dilutes, so Frog Clan people have an ability to discern emotional blockages in others and to help to dissolve them. They can also dilute any build-up of negative energies which can often lead to physical, mental and emotional sickness. However, less positively, Frog Clan people can cause emotional blockages in themselves which can have a devastating effect on the flow of vital energies within themselves and within those who are closest to them.

The motivating force of the Frog Clan is the need to develop and mature.

4.7 Birth and Animal Totem: Woodpecker

The totem animal of those born in the Long Days Time is the Woodpecker – a colourful bird with a strong, sharp beak which is able to chip away at branches and tree trunks to create a nesting chamber or to bore in to catch insects.

The Woodpecker was specially regarded by the Amerindian because the rhythm of its pecking was similar to that of the shaman's drum simulating the human heartbeat or the natural rhythm of the pulse of the Earth itself. And Woodpeckers were observed to perform their drumming, not always out of the necessity for food or shelter, but for sheer enjoyment and this particularly endeared them to the Indian.

The Woodpecker has sharp claws which enable it to cling to trees while it performs its drumming, and like their animal totem, Woodpecker people are inclined to cling tenaciously to things, and even to people.

Like the bird, Woodpecker people make good parents, too, but have difficulty in letting go of their young ones when they are old enough to make their own way in the world and will cling on to them even into old age, making their offspring continue to feel dependent on them. 'Letting go' is one of the hardest experiences for Woodpecker people to undertake for it is, in fact, a test of true love.

Just as Woodpeckers make a comfortable nest for themselves and for their young, so Woodpecker people require a comfortable and harmonious home. Indeed, the home and the close relationships it entails are absolutely vital for their well-being. If they are unable to share their 'nest' with someone they love, Woodpecker people – particularly women – can become bitter and even twisted.

Woodpeckers need someone or something to serve, to direct their energies and devotion towards. If they lack the means to channel their devotion, then they become very unhappy and wallow in a pool of negative emotions.

4.8 PLANT TOTEM: Wild rose

There are many species of the wild rose, which is a prickly shrub with trailing, climbing or erect stems. It produces five-petalled pinkish, reddish or white flowers. After the flowers disappear, fruit-like hips are formed and these are orange-coloured when ripe. The flowers blossom from May until July, and the hips are ready for harvesting in the autumn.

The wild rose has many medicinal properties. Dried rose petals can be taken for headaches and, mixed with honey, as a tonic and blood-purifier. Rose-water made from the petals was used by Amerindians as eye lotion and for relieving discomfort for hay fever sufferers. Rose petals were also made into an oil and used as a perfume. Dried petals also made a pleasant air-freshener.

Rosehips are rich in Vitamin C and are a fine remedy for colds, sore throats and influenza.

Like their plant totem, people born at this time can bring beauty, harmony and freshness into the lives of others, though they can be overly protective towards their offspring, and they do have a prickly side to their nature.

4.9 MINERAL TOTEM: Rose quartz

Rose quartz is a crystalline quartz whose delicate pink colour is due to traces of manganese. It is a stone which works with the heart chakra and I am told that it makes a person receptive to beautiful things – not just by enhancing an appreciation of beauty in physical objects, but of sounds (music), colours (art) and forms (poetry).

Since it harmonizes with the heart chakra, rose quartz helps to dissolve traumas, sorrows, fears and resentments that burden the heart, and it promotes understanding. It is a stone that is both a transmitter and a receiver, so it should be carried on the person.

It is said to encourage love between parents and children and has the attribute of strengthening family unity and kinship.

People of this totem develop strong family relationships and show a willingness to sacrifice much for the happiness of their children. Rose quartz is reputed to promote friendship and to disperse anger and strife.

Rose quartz is a healing stone and a helpful support in times of emergency. Similarly, Woodpecker people are helpful in emergencies, and with their intuitive insight are often able to know just what is required to deal with a sudden crisis situation.

4.10 POLARITY TOTEM: Goose

Woodpeckers' intense feelings cause them to be protective towards their loved ones, but they can be overly protective and so unbalanced that they can turn their home into a prison.

Woodpeckers can learn from their polar opposite, Goose, to widen their horizon beyond the influence of the home, and to seek ways to serve those who are outside their family or clan. Woodpeckers need to develop outside interests and to engage in absorbing hobbies or sporting pursuits.

Because Woodpeckers live so often on raw, emotional energy, they need to acquire discipline and self-control, and Goose can teach them that. They must learn, too, not to harp on the past and 'what might have been', otherwise their life will be filled with regrets. Goose can show them how to balance their energies more effectively.

4.11 PERSONALITY EXPRESSION
Adult

Emotional, sensitive, protective and vulnerable. Woodpecker people have a strong paternal or maternal instinct. Their lives centre around the home, which is the only place they really feel safe in, and around their own family. They are warm and loving to those who are closest to them, but show a hard exterior to strangers.

They are highly emotional and easily upset. Indeed they will often play on the sympathy and loyalty of loved ones by appearing emotionally deprived and neglected, often magnifying a situation out of all proportion.

They develop strong attachments and will cling to whatever is important to them with a never-let-go tenacity. In fact, it is attachments that cause them the most stress and anxiety and even sickness. Through life-experiences, they must learn detachment in order to take control of their lives.

They are natural worriers, and their powerful imagination can often run riot so they become overly concerned about the future instead of getting on with the present.

Woodpecker people can swing between two extremes. They can be warm, kind and considerate on the one hand, and harsh, moody and bitter on the other.

Positive traits: Sensitive. Imaginative. Sympathetic. Protective. Tender. Shrewd. Thrifty.

Negative traits: Over-emotional. Hypersensitive. Moody. Unforgiving. Untidy.

Vocational possibilities: Art. Banking. Civil law. Consultancy work. Import/export. Nursing. Navy. Perfumery. Property. Theatre. Priesthood.

Child

The Woodpecker child is generally quite happy to play by itself without demanding constant attention, and is one of the easiest to bring up. It seems to enjoy its own company, and its active imagination helps it to find its own amusement.

Woodpecker children are sensitive though, and easily hurt. A harsh word can have a devastating effect and send them into a dark cloud of moodiness. They develop excellent memories, which enables them to absorb information easily. They are also good at soaking up the opinions of others and regurgitating them as their own.

Parent

Woodpeckers make caring parents and take great pleasure in their children. It seems that their sensitive nature is responsive to the vulnerability and innocence of a child.

Woodpecker fathers are proud, protective and patient, and Woodpecker mothers so caring that there is a tendency to overdo their protectiveness and to pamper their offspring. The Woodpecker mother is often reluctant to let her children grow up, and still regards them as her 'babies' sometimes long after they have children of their own.

4.12 ROMANCE AND SEX

Woodpecker people like to be held and cuddled and dealt with tenderly. They enjoy caressing and being caressed, and are turned on by kissing – particularly the slow, lingering kind. They are so highly charged emotionally that once they give their heart their commitment is total.

The male Woodpecker, however, has a need that requires more emotional than physical satisfaction. It may be that he is looking more for a mother than a wife.

The female Woodpecker has a more assertive sexual appetite. Indeed, it could be said of her that sex is as important to her as food – and she likes her food.

Woodpeckers are easily hurt, and disappointment, frustration or just plain denial can lead them to adopt a woe-is-me, nobody-loves-me attitude to life.

Though Woodpeckers can be kind and affable, thoughtful and understanding, they can swing to the other extreme and be bad-tempered, irritable, moody and snappy. At times they may be sympathetic and understanding towards their partner's problems, and at other times concerned only with their own often exaggerated woes when any tiny hurt can be magnified into a great injustice and the topic of constant harping.

Compatibilities: Woodpeckers are compatible with Snakes, Wolves and Beavers (those born between 23 October and 22 November, 19 February and 20 March, and 20 April and 20 May).

Spiritual sexuality: (–) The basic spiritual sexuality of Woodpeckers is feminine, but of course this is not referring to gender. It means that they are usually introverted, nurturing and protective. Woodpeckers' emotional receptivity makes them especially vulnerable and easily hurt.

4.13 HEALTH

Woodpecker people are generally robust and quick to recover from most illnesses. They are, however, sensitive to pain and have a low pain-resistance threshold.

Their weak areas are the chest and breasts and the stomach. They are prone to bronchial infections and stomach disorders. Invariably stomach upsets are brought on by worry.

4.14 AFFINITY COLOUR: Rose

Rose is a deeper colour than pink, partaking more of the energy of red, and it works with the emotions. It is particularly helpful to Woodpecker people as a balancer and a guard against moodiness and extremes.

Like its flower counterpart, it is associated with the affections and sentiments, for rose is the colour of compassion and of bringing together. It also signifies the desire to serve. Its attribute is loving-kindness which is the quality Woodpecker people need as a balancer of their inner dynamics.

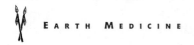

Woodpeckers should find that wearing something rose-coloured, whether it is an item of clothing or an accessory, or even a handkerchief, brooch or tiepin, will have a beneficial effect on the way they feel and that they are not so emotionally vulnerable.

4.15 ADVANTAGEOUS TIMES

Best months of the year for Woodpecker people are from 21 June to 22 July, 23 October to 22 November, and from 19 February to 20 March.
Best day of the week is Monday.
Best times of the day are from 9 a.m. to 11 a.m. and 9 p.m. to 11 p.m.

4.16 OUTWARD (CONSCIOUS) AIM AND INNER (SUBCONSCIOUS) DESIRE

Outwardly, Woodpeckers seem driven to express themselves primarily through their feelings. The problem is that this emotional expression often leads them to feel vulnerable.

Inwardly, there is a desire to know the right time to act, the right time to hold on and the right time to let go, and this leads them to feel unsure and insecure.

Woodpeckers' attitudes are so often shaped by their past experiences, and especially those incidents when they feel threatened or inadequate. They hold on to these as if they happened only yesterday, and as a consequence have a tendency to harbour grievances for a very long time. Although sympathetic by nature, Woodpeckers can be unforgiving towards people they feel have threatened their security or brought their inadequacy to the surface in the past.

Reconciliation of the outer and inner expressions comes when Woodpeckers learn to let go of the past and let bygones be bygones. The purpose of this apparent conflict is for them to learn to cope with change through adaptation. When that happens they will free their creativity from the boundaries of self-imposed limitations and set if free through outlets where it can also help others. Then their own personal security will be ensured.

4.17 SPIRITUAL ALCHEMY

With so much emphasis on elemental Water, Woodpecker people live on their emotions. They feel so deeply that they often suffer the emotional traumas of other people, especially members of their own family. It is essential, therefore, that they get to understand their emotions and not

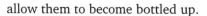

allow them to become bottled up.

Just as water finds its own level and adjusts to the surroundings it is in, so Woodpecker people must learn to adjust, not just to physical environment but to the people they are brought into contact with.

Since the south-south-east direction indicates the movement from warm to hot it is represented by two yang (=) or (+ +). Elemental Water is an influence both in its directional and cyclical activity (– –). The spiritual sexuality of Woodpecker is feminine (–). So the combination of these essential factors is (+ +, – – and –) which indicates a personality that is more passive than outgoing and is protective.

4.18 LIFE-CHALLENGES

Woodpeckers are born worriers and can see doom and disaster as the outcome of almost any situation. They worry about how a situation might end almost before it has begun.

Part of their life-purpose is to discover how to live in the Now. Every experience in life is endeavouring to teach them the importance of treasuring the moment.

Woodpeckers need to cultivate their intuitiveness and resourcefulness and to come to recognize the healing balm of forgiveness. They need to avoid self-pity, recrimination, feeling sorry for themselves, and harbouring envy. But the quality they need to let go of the most is their possessiveness.

4.19 PRIMARY FUNCTION AND LIFE-PATH

The primary function of Woodpecker is to assimilate experience through the feelings and to draw knowledge and wisdom from them. By so doing, emotional unfoldment is obtained.

The path Woodpeckers are on leads towards the recognition that love has a polarity of its own and has to be given to be received and to be released in order to be retained, and if held by the grip of possessiveness becomes stifled and suffocates.

The emphasis is on total commitment and a need to accept trials and difficulties, conflicts and even defeats, as necessary experiences if one is to emerge a stronger personality. The greatest difficulty on this path is in learning to handle one's own contradictions, and harnessing the powers that are within.

The prime purpose, then, is to harness the turbulent, instinctive and emotional nature and to bring it under the control of the will in order to attain true maturity.

4.20 THE I CHING TRIGRAM: **Tui. The Joyous Lake.**

Those born in the Long Days Time are on the south-south-east direction on the Wheel of the Year and share the same trigram as those of the previous time on the south-east direction.

The Joyous Lake represents the desire for contentment, which is very strong in Woodpecker people. It is the joy of satisfaction – the satisfaction of physical love, the satisfaction that comes from achievement, and the satisfaction of attainment and of work well done.

4.21 HOW TO COPE WITH WOODPECKERS

Handle them gently. They are highly emotional and changeable and will withdraw into themselves if they think they and anyone or anything that 'belongs' to them is being threatened.

By positive in their company. You may feel better yourself after relating your troubles, but Woodpecker is inclined to be so sympathetic that your worries become their own. Woodpeckers catch worries as easily as some people catch colds.

Don't try to push Woodpeckers too hard. They will be led, but they won't be driven.

Salmon

SUMMARY

Birth dates:	22 July – 21 August (20 January – 18 February in the Southern hemisphere).
Earth influence:	The Ripening Time.
Influencing wind:	South Winds. *Totem:* Mouse.
Direction:	South.
Predominant elements:	Fire with Water.
Elemental clan:	Hawk (Fire) Clan. *Function:* to do.
Birth and animal totem:	Salmon.
Plant totem:	Raspberry.
Mineral totem:	Carnelian.
Polarity totem:	Otter.
Affinity colour:	Red.
Personality:	Proud. Energetic. Confident. Enthusiastic.
Feelings:	Passionate. Intense.
Intention:	Rulership.
Nature:	Demanding.
Positive traits:	Generous. Magnanimous. Creative.
Negative traits:	Domineering. Arrogant. Dogmatic. Intolerant.
Sex-drive:	Insatiable.
Compatibilities:	Owls and Falcons.
Conscious aim:	To rule.
Subconscious desire:	Emotional stability.
Life-path:	To find purpose.
I Ching trigram:	☵ K'an. Water. Desire for consistency.
Spiritual alchemy:	Yang predominates.
Must cultivate:	Tolerance. Sound judgement. Emotional stability.
Must avoid:	Arrogance. Egotism, Pomposity. Indolence.
Starting totems:	Salmon. Mouse. Hawk, Raspberry. Carnelian. Otter.

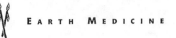

5. Salmon

5.1 BIRTH MONTH: 22 July – 21 August

5.2 EARTH INFLUENCE: The Ripening Time

The month from 22 July to 21 August is the period when the Sun is at its hottest in the Northern hemisphere and ripens the fruits of the Earth. It is a time when, traditionally, we pause from our labours to bask in the sunshine and to refresh ourselves before the work of harvesting which is to come. It is the time when the whole of Nature appears to be opening up to the Sun and bringing forth its fruit in abundance.

The Ripening Time was thus regarded as a time of openness and warmth and these qualities are reflected in those people whose birthdays occur at this time.

Half-way through this month occurred a Fire festival of the old religions of Northern Europe which was called Lammas, and by the Celts, Lughnasadh. It was held on 1 August and in Britain was sometimes called 'the Feast of the First Fruits!' It marked the first cut of harvest corn while summer was still in full swing and was the season of fairs. It recognized that after the Summer Solstice the Sun had begun to wane and its power was declining.

Although it was a joyous, happy time it served also as a reminder that all is not as it might appear. For though the Sun was shining and the days were hot, the Circle was beginning to dip towards the dark and the days were shortening in preparation for the autumn and the approach of winter.

It was, then, a festival of reminder – a reminder that things are not always as they may appear, and that nothing in the physical world is permanent.

And it was a time for reflection – a reminder of what we are now and what we hope to become.

5.3 SOLAR INFLUENCES

This month is the peak of the summer power with the animating life-force of the Sun reaching maturity and causing bountiful activity. It is the time when the heat of the Sun ripens the fruits of the Earth.

Those born during this month when the Sun is at its most powerful are usually energetic and creative with an outgoing personality and a temperament which could be described as 'sunny'.

The influence of the solar energies on their ego is evident in their self-esteem for, like the Sun, they like being looked up to and appreciated. The related sign in Sun astrology is Leo.

5.4 INFLUENCING WIND: South Winds
DIRECTION: South

The warm south winds bring a flow of vital energies to those born in the Ripening Time that gives them a capacity to take on difficult tasks which others might decline, and to accept the burden of responsibility. It is this primal energy that makes them so active and energetic and bold and determined leaders who enjoy the excitement of being out in front.

The totem animal of the South is *mouse*. For people who can be as bold, aggressive and dominant as those born in the Ripening Time to be influenced by tiny Mouse, may seem ridiculous. But as was stated in the precious section under 4.4, we must not underestimate the value of little Mouse.

Mouse is associated with comprehending things by being close to them. It is especially related to the emotions and feelings, and with the qualities of trust and innocence.

A full explanation is given in section 4.4.

The emphasis in the Ripening Time is especially on the need to trust one's feelings and intuitions during the pain of change which will be experienced during the process of maturing.

5.5 INFLUENCING ELEMENTS: Fire with Water

Elemental Water is the influence of the directional power of the South and, as we learned in the previous section (4.5), is concerned with the emotions and feelings.

But water is also a 'mixing' agent – a means of changing through dissolving and diluting – so it also has to do with transformation.

The change which elemental Water is bringing about in those born during the Ripening Time is not instant, but is a process which takes time. People of this month will have an urge to push ahead and to bring about desired changes, but they will still want to retain that which has been tried and tested. Primarily, it is likely to be the family that they will look to as their anchor and their security.

Elemental Fire is the influence of the cyclical power and it is this influence which makes them activators and trail-blazers and full of zest.

5.6 ELEMENTAL CLAN: **The Hawk (Fire) Clan**

People born during the Ripening Time come under the Hawk Clan, which is the clan of elemental Fire. Elemental Fire causes them to be outgoing and energetic with an insatiable inner drive to be always doing something. Such individuals are usually at the hub of any activity in which they are involved. They are so full of zest that they are in danger of burning themselves out through their intensity and over-zealousness and lack of caution.

They like the warmth that comes from close relationships, and they like to have bright things around them. The decor of their homes is usually warm and bright. This affinity with the Sun and elemental Fire can be used beneficially by them in times of need. For instance, when they feel wound up through the intensity of their activities, or they feel drained and in need of replenishment, a bask in the Sun, a relaxing session in a solarium, watching the flames in a campfire or fireplace, or just gazing into the flame of a candle, can have a remarkably soothing effect and quickly restore them to balance.

Hawk Clan people have an inner radiance and a fiery temperament, and should familiarize themselves with the Sun in its phases and seasons for it can help them to understand their own temperament and to learn how to temper and control their own inner light. (See also 1.6 and 9.6.)

5.7 BIRTH AND ANIMAL TOTEM: **Salmon**

In Britain and northern Europe in ancient times the Salmon was regarded as the King of the Fishes. The salmon is a magnificent creature that can grow to a length of up to 120 cm (4 ft) and weigh over 30 kg (66 lb). It displays an amazing feat of navigational skill as it finds its way from the sea to the river of its birth and swims upstream to its spawning grounds. In this journey it can leap waterfalls up to 3 metres (10 ft) high.

Perhaps because of this tremendous achievement, the salmon in legendary tales was said to swim in waters of inspiration and foreknowledge, and was thus associated with wisdom and with strength of purpose.

A similar fish, the sturgeon, was used as a totem among many American Indian tribes. It, too, moves between sea and fresh water, living in the muddy bottoms of estuaries and moving upstream to more shallow waters to spawn in the spring. Its skin is very tough, and it has rows of bony plates which makes it the armoured knight of the waters.

The sturgeon was regarded by the Amerindians as the Keeper of Longevity because it could survive to a ripe old age. Potentially, people who have sturgeon or salmon as a totem are blessed with longevity in order that they shall learn to grow old gracefully.

The movement of salmon and sturgeon through the water is so graceful that the fish cause almost no disturbance. People born in the Ripening Time should emulate their totem animal and learn to move through life without creating friction and disturbance, for it is their resistance to change and the demands that others put upon them that causes most of their emotional upsets.

Since Water is related to the emotions and the salmon is such a master of the water, the lessons of life for Salmon people are to teach them to attain mastery of their emotions.

5.8 PLANT TOTEM: Raspberry

The raspberry (*Rubus strigosus*) is a tall, woody plant that grows cane-like up to 150 cm (5 ft) tall and whose leaves are light green with pale undersides. It blossoms in May with white cup-shaped flowers, and the berries ripen in July. The berries are made up of globe-shaped segments, each of which grows around its own pip.

The berries are delicious and of considerable medicinal value for they cleanse the system, act as a mild laxative, and stimulate the urinary organs.

The root of the plant is astringent and has antibiotic properties. The leaves can be used to make a mild and pleasant herbal tea which is said to relieve nausea, especially in pregnant women, and can also be helpful during times of menstruation. It helps to cleanse the mucous membranes, and also balances the blood sugar levels.

Like their plant totem, Salmon people are often sought out by others for enjoyment. Like the fruit of the raspberry, Salmon people are not what they appear to be. The fruit appears to be a berry but is, in fact an aggregate of a number of small, separate drupes. Salmon people might appear to be hard and even callous because of their courageousness, but under the surface there is a warm and soft heart. Or they may appear charming and affectionate and even soft-hearted, but can have a prickly interior.

Like the raspberry, Salmon people can be helpful for those around them to get their problems out of their systems.

5.9 MINERAL TOTEM: Carnelian

Carnelian is a translucent to clear chalcedony, a smooth, waxy form of quartz which is found in rock cavities. It is flesh-coloured, or red, orange or reddish-brown. Its name means 'flesh-coloured'.

It is the stone of integrity and among Indians was often a symbol of strength and beauty of the Earth.

Carnelian has a subtle, vibrant quality and was, therefore, attributed with the ability to stimulate and to stir into action. I am told that it softens anger and disperses strife – conditions which are frequently experienced by Salmon people – and promotes contentment, so it is a stone they should carry or wear.

Since Salmon people are usually intense individuals with a tendency to dominate others and to act impulsively, Carnelian can help them to develop self-control.

It is a stone of blood ties and family unity since its principal attribute is to strengthen.

Amerindians credited the Carnelian with curative powers and it was used in general healing. It was sometimes suspended on a thong and used as a pendulum above a wound and its circular movement was said to start the healing process.

5.10 POLARITY TOTEM: Otter

Salmon's outgoing temperament and desire for action can lead them into impulsive actions which result in misunderstandings that hurt their inner sensitivity.

They can guard against this by learning from their polar opposite, Otter, which, although considered one of the most noble of animals is also most playful. Otter can serve as an example to Salmon to balance their intensity with periods of playful relaxation, and to temper their aggressive-ness with gentleness.

Salmon can learn from Otter to discover for themselves that there is strength in gentleness, and that there is a power in compassion that can bring about desirable changes.

True attainment often comes from letting go, and remembering also that getting is a partner of giving. Otter points the way to the recognition of such truths.

5.11 PERSONALITY EXPRESSION
Adult

There are no half measures about proud, energetic, enthusiastic Salmon. Confidence oozes from them. Not only will they leave no doubt that they should be running things, but that they're able to run other people's lives also. Such arrogance is expressed in so warm-hearted a manner that others are inclined to let them get on with it.

Salmon people are just as uncompromising in their opinions. Whatever view they hold at the moment is the only right one. The snag is that they are inclined to change their views quite radically, but they will promote their latest opinion with such fervour and conviction that they'll convince others it's the only one they ever had. Their air of self-importance is coupled with a thirst for personal glory and an appetite for self-assertion, but emotionally they are vulnerable, easily hurt by neglect or withdrawal of love.

Although they are quite rational it is difficult for Salmon to make balanced judgements because their egotistical nature makes them vulnerable to flattery and deceit. They love to dramatize and as a result will often inflate problems and situations out of all proportion.

The male Salmon is good at fixing things, whether it is something in the home that won't work or has come apart, or whether it is a situation in someone else's life. They are experts at telling people how to run their lives, but they clock up quite a few problems in endeavouring to manage their own.

Although he has an optimistic outlook, he is likely to crumble under the weight of gloom and despondency if he is overtaken by adversity, crossed in love, or betrayed by someone close to him.

The female Salmon is concerned about her appearance and will be fastidious about the clothes she wears. She makes a loyal friend, but her judgements of people are not always sound. She is too easily deceived by appearances or by flattering words, rather than measuring others by their worth of character and their warmth of personality.

Both male and female Salmon take great care about how they look, almost to the point of vanity. The male Salmon will be aware of his physique and his fitness, the female about her clothes, her hair-do and especially her make-up.

Positive traits: Generous. Magnanimous. Creative. Enthusiastic. Trusting. Authoritative. Proud.

Negative traits: Domineering. Arrogant. Vain. Immodest. Dogmatic. Intolerant. Pompous.

Vocational possibilities: Arts. Administrative work. Films. Television. Public Relations. Psychology. Politics. Newspaper work. Military. Show business. Theology.

Child

The Salmon baby revels in attention, especially the adoring kind. The more fuss that's made of the little one, the happier it becomes. Indeed, watch an infant Salmon in its cot surrounded by doting parents and admirers and it simply exudes happiness.

The Salmon infant is playful and jolly so long as it gets what it wants – and it generally wants attention more than things. But continue to spoil the Salmon baby into childhood and you could have a little tyrant on your hands. If little Salmon is to grow up respecting the rights of others as well as having respect for itself, it is likely to need the application of some gentle discipline and clear guidance from time to time, and be made to realize that it is not the only child in the world.

Salmon children and quick to learn, but tend to be lazy, so they may need encouragement. Challenge them to show they can do better than the others!

Parent

Salmon folk make proud and affectionate parents, though they risk being too authoritarian and may tend to rule their children to the point of stifling their personalities and denying them self-reliance. Salmon fathers in particular want to stamp their own personality on their offspring.

Salmon do not find parenthood burdensome. Indeed, they tackle it with enthusiasm, and spend time with their children, deriving a great deal of happiness and satisfaction from the experience.

5.12 ROMANCE AND SEX

Love is essential to the well-being of Salmon people. The male Salmon is a warm, intense and demonstrative lover. The female Salmon has a captivating charm and is rather theatrical in expressing her emotions.

Salmon give themselves totally. They are capable of making mad, passionate love, and are so energetic that they can keep going through the night.

As a husband, the male Salmon is a good provider. He might resent having a career girl as a wife – and even more so if her job is more responsible or financially more rewarding than his. As far as he is concerned, *he* is his wife's career!

The sex-drive of the female Salmon is strong and she needs love constantly to remain well-balanced.

Compatibilities: Salmon are compatible with Owls and Falcons (those born between 23 November and 21 December and 21 March and 19 April).

Spiritual sexuality: (+) The basic spiritual sexuality of Salmon is masculine, which means they are usually extroverted, thrusting and energetic.

5.13 HEALTH

Salmon are rarely ill and when they are they have good recuperative powers. It is the intensity of their activities that is likely to cause health problems. Because they don't know their own limitations or recognize their emotional vulnerability, they run the risk of overdoing things and as a consequence may suffer from stress disorders. High blood-pressure is likely as they get older, and other problems may develop from impaired circulation.

Their tendency to push themselves hard makes them prone to injuries, especially to the back, and to fractures of the legs or ankles.

5.14 AFFINITY COLOUR: Red

The red ray, with the longest and slowest wavelength in the spectrum, is related more to the physical aspect. Red is enlivening and stimulating, and is the colour that gets the adrenalin going and perks up the nervous system.

People influenced by red are usually assertive and want their own way without restraint. They are individualistic and want to assert themselves and the beliefs they hold.

Red's purpose might be described as expression through external experiences. It provides an impulse to win, but those affected by it usually perceive only objectives. So Salmon people enjoy being engaged in a whirlwind of activity, but should their avenues of expression and expansion be blocked in any way, they are likely to become frustrated and anxious and suffer the effects of nervous tension.

Salmon people are likely to show extremes of behaviour, and be domineering and aggressive, and passionate in their attitudes and actions. It is hard to achieve balance and tolerance of the ideas and beliefs of others when the red ray is such a powerful influence, but that is the big lesson to be learned by Salmon through their life experiences.

Periods of relaxation which do not required the expenditure of large amounts of physical energy, and times set aside for quiet reflection and meditation, are the routes towards finding that balance.

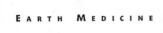

5.15 Advantageous Times
Best months of the year for Salmon people are from 22 July to 21 August,
23 November to 21 December and 21 March to 19 April.
Best day of the week is Sunday.
Best times of the day are from 11 a.m. to 1 p.m. and 11 p.m. to 1 a.m.

5.16 Outward (Conscious) Aim and Inner (Subconscious) Desire
The Salmon's outward aim is rulership. Salmon must have their own way,
otherwise they are overcome by their greatest fear – the fear of failure.

The inner desire is for the gaining of wisdom on the emotional plane, for
although Salmon have strong hearts on the physical level, they have a weakness emotionally. Their inner quest is motivated by a subconscious desire to
rectify the emotional vulnerability which is their greatest weakness.

5.17 Spiritual Alchemy
The intensity and transmuting qualities that come through the influence of
elemental Fire are counteracted by the emotional sensitivity that comes
through elemental Water. It indicates that growth comes through the
experience of close relationships and the lessons of being touched by
emotional unfoldment. The Fire of change is brought into contact with the
Water of the emotions for the purpose of bringing about an elevation of
the desires and intentions which rise above and beyond the mundane.
With a very active directional influence (+ +), the elemental polarities of
Fire (+) and Water (–), and masculine spirituality (+), the personality is
thus aggressively masculine. The combination is thus (+ +, + – and +).

5.18 Life-Challenges
Salmon are likely to find themselves in life-situations in which it is
necessary for them to discover how to heal their emotional hurts and to
escape from a seemingly endless cycle of emotional upsets and traumas
without losing their compassion, warm-heartedness and capacity to love
and be loved.

Learning to move through the waters of emotion without creating
resistance is one of the principal challenges of their lives, for it is resistance
to change and disregard of the emotional needs of others which causes
them their greatest traumas and upsets.

Must cultivate: Tolerance. Sound judgement. Emotional stability.
Must avoid: Arrogance. Pomposity. Egotism. Indolence.

5.19 PRIMARY FUNCTION AND LIFE-PATH

The primary function of Salmon might be described as the acquisition of distinctive individual character, which they are constantly seeking to express. But the life-path leads towards something more than that.

Salmon's desire to be the centre of attention stems from their need to stand out from the crowd and thereby establish their individuality. Although they are equipped with a strong will to enable them to push themselves forward, they are in need of constant reassurance in order to maintain their self-esteem.

The path they are on is to lead them to discover purposefulness. But that can only be found when they use their intrinsic strengths of will and commitment not to overpower and lord it over others, but in the direction of a chosen purposeful goal. Their life-path is likely to lead them into making things happen by the use of the will and not by 'using' others. It is power and rulership over experiences that is the strength they require to obtain with the strengths they have been given. The discovery and use of that is the purpose of Salmon's life. Learning to control one's own ferocious egotism requires the development of great strength – not the exertion of physical power, but the spiritual strength which alone can control the more difficult aspects of the human psyche.

Salmon's prime purpose is the ability to put trust and integrity in place of pride and vanity, and for Salmon that is no easy task.

5.20 THE I CHING TRIGRAM: K'an. The Abysmal Water.

Those born in the Ripening Time are on the South direction on the Wheel of the Year. The Abysmal Water trigram represents the uncertainty of deep and dangerous water. It is perilous to all except those who have learned to swim well.

One cannot stand still in fast-flowing water because it is in a constant state of rapid motion. Consistency comes through being true to the Inner Self because there is an infinite intelligence within that knows and that will respond once it is recognized. That is where stillness lies.

5.21 HOW TO COPE WITH SALMON

Get to the point quickly. Salmon don't like hanging about. Listen to Salmon's point of view – it is the only one that counts to them. They get impatient with people who interrupt them.

Encourage Salmon through praise, but not flattery. If Salmon suspects you are insincere you'll fast lose their respect.

Brown Bear

SUMMARY

Birth dates:	22 August – 21 September (19 February – 20 March in the Southern hemisphere).
Earth influence:	The Harvesting Time.
Influencing wind:	The South Winds. *Totem*: Mouse.
Direction:	South-south-west.
Predominant elements:	Earth with Water.
Elemental clan:	Turtle (Earth) Clan. *Function*: to modify.
Birth and animal totem:	Brown Bear.
Plant totem:	Violets.
Mineral totem:	Topaz.
Polarity totem:	Wolf.
Affinity colour:	Brown and violet.
Personality:	Industrious. Unassuming. Practical. Fastidious.
Feelings:	Warm. Analytical.
Intention:	Practicality.
Nature:	Considerate.
Positive traits:	Modest. Discriminating. Meticulous.
Negative traits:	Fault-finding. Finicky. Hypocritical. Fussy.
Sex-drive:	Moralistic.
Compatibilities:	Geese and Beavers.
Conscious aim:	Sifting and striving.
Subconscious desire:	Perfection.
Life-path:	Discrimination.
I Ching trigram:	⚎ Chen. Arousing Thunder. ▬ Desire for liberation.
Spiritual alchemy:	Yin predominates.
Must cultivate:	Optimism. Tolerance.
Must avoid:	Scepticism. Fault-finding. Procrastination.
Starting totems:	Brown Bear. Mouse. Turtle. Violet. Topaz. Wolf.

6. Brown Bear

6.1 BIRTH MONTH: 22 August – 21 September

6.2 EARTH INFLUENCE: The Harvesting Time

The Harvesting Time marks the time for reaping what has been sown and for drawing in from the Earth's bounty, though it has much more significance than the harvesting of produce. For people born during this month it stresses the importance of harvesting the potentialities that lie within. It indicates the need to discover one's talents and to work on them so that they can be brought to their full potential. It is a reminder, too, that one gets from life in proportion to what one puts in.

6.3 SOLAR INFLUENCES

The peak of the summer power has now passed as the solar energies wane towards another transition in the seasonal cycle and the days shorten.

The emphasis of the solar energies at this time is on the immediate and practical work that is at hand, for there is an urgency about the gathering in as well as a responsibility, for neglect can lead to deprivation in times to come.

The related sign in Sun astrology is Virgo.

6.4 INFLUENCING WIND: South Winds
DIRECTION: South-south-west

The Harvesting Time is the last cycle under the influence of the Spirit of the South, whose emphasis is on trust and on growth to maturity. The trust, as we have seen in the two earlier cycles of the South, is a childlike dependence on one's own inherent instincts and on that still, small voice within as against the cynicism and false values of the 'outside' world.

The growth to maturity also implies retaining the quality of innocence which is so strongly emphasized in the South – an innocence which does not mean naivity but a state of non-attachment, and which sees not differences but the unity that is in the harmony of a whole. Trust and innocence, as understood by the Amerindian, enriched the experience of living through the enjoyment of life's simple pleasures.

Under this time, the quality of trust is a guard against becoming too cynical and too critical about the world and the circumstances of one's life, and the quality of growth is a prod against becoming too rigid in one's outlook on life and too set in one's ways.

Growth to the fullness of maturity and to a subsequent reaching upwards to the things of the spirit, can take place only if the earth energies are firmly grounded. The influence of the power of the South is towards the harvesting of the fruits of practical endeavours while at the same time allowing the intuitive and spiritual energies to develop and in this way allowing an expansion of awareness that is beyond that which is physical.

The totem animal of the South is *mouse*, which is associated with comprehending things through closeness to them. It is especially related to the feelings and emotions and with the qualities of trust and innocence. Turn back to section 4.4 for a fuller explanation.

Harvesting Time people need to involve desire and feeling in their practical endeavours in order to enhance the quality of that which is harvested from them.

6.5 INFLUENCING ELEMENTS: Earth with Water

Water is not just a superb solvent which can absorb and dissolve harmful impurities. It is a great container, able to hold within its grasp the substance that is poured into it.

Water is likened to the emotions which are also able to absorb and dissolve negative influences and dilute them so they cause no permanent harm. The emotions are also able to contain the essence of powerful spiritual qualities which are awaiting to be expressed in accordance with the will and desire.

Elemental Water is a powerful influence for Harvesting Time people because it can help to bring into fruition practical endeavours that have been mixed with strong feelings and desire. It is also through the waters of emotion that the innermost desires of Harvesting Time people can find expression to the elevation of themselves and those with whom the emotion is being shared.

In addition, Harvesting Time people are affected by Elemental Earth, which gives them a close affinity with the Earth and with familiar places. It means they thrive best in settled, stable and harmonious environments.

6.6 ELEMENTAL CLAN: Turtle (Earth) Clan

Harvesting Time people are related to the Turtle Clan, which is the influence of Elemental Earth. People of this clan feel a need to put down roots and to have a stable base from which to operate, and they like to have solid and familiar things around them. They resent dramatic and sudden change.

It is the Earth Element in their make-up that enables them to make progress carefully and through the application of persistence and tenacity.

They have a solidity that makes them loyal and dependable friends, workmates or business associates, and a staying power that enables them to swim through the waters of adversity and find a firm footing afterwards.

They have a close affinity with Nature, and enjoy tending the Earth and growing things. They feel drawn to places where there are hills or mountains.

6.7 BIRTH AND ANIMAL TOTEM: Brown Bear

The brown bear can grow to $1^1/_2$ metres (4 or 5 ft) in length, and weigh up to 18 kg (400 lb) and though they have enormous strength they are amongst the gentlest of animals and their behaviour can be almost 'human'. They can walk on two legs, climb trees like a human, and even catch fish with their paws. They are generally good-natured animals unless trapped or threatened. They have a growl or bark like a dog.

The brown bear makes its den in caves or behind waterfalls, and sometimes in holes or derelict buildings. It will eat almost anything – grass, plants, berries, nuts, vegetables, fish and small animals. It is particularly fond of honey and berries.

Bears hibernate in winter, though they sometimes awaken on a warm day to venture outside their den. Bear cubs are born in early spring and are raised by the mother. It takes about seven years for a bear to grow to maturity.

Like their animal totems, Brown Bear people are self-reliant and prefer to stand on their own two feet rather than rely on others. They take time to acclimatize to change, preferring the security and comfort of the familiar. They are constructive and good fixers, with an innate ability to get things working, whether in dealing with the break-down of a piece of equipment or in human relations where they are often able to contribute their 'mending' balm of tenderness and understanding.

The Amerindian regarded the Brown Bear as a dreamer, and like their totem animal Brown Bear people, though endowed with practical skills, are essentially dreamers. Their imagination enables them to see clearly a situation they would like to be in and they can be so carried away by the daydream that they become almost convinced of its physical reality. As a result they are sometimes accused of lying.

6.8 Plant Totem: Violets

Violets (*viola*) are small, distinctive, perennial plants that grow in woodland and grassland. Some species flower earlier than other spring flowers. The dark green leaves are heart-shaped. The five-petalled flowers in the more common varieties are violet colour or blue-violet. The creeping rootstock sends out runners along the ground and these also take root.

Medicinally, the leaves were used to make a soothing gargle for sore throats, and the rootstock was used to make a syrup remedy for coughs. The dried leaves, used as a tea, soothed stomach and bowel disorders.

Possibly because of its distinctive fragrance, the violet is associated with warm and tender sentiments. Like their plant totem, Brown Bear people express the warmth of their sentiments through close-to-the-ground practical actions.

Like the violet, Brown Bear people have an aloof nature. They do not inflict themselves on others, or interfere in others' lives. But their aloofness can sometimes cause them to suffer loneliness.

6.9 Mineral Totem: Topaz

Topaz is an aluminium fluorine silicate found in granite and other indigenous rocks. The soft, golden brown topaz is a delicate stone but it has great strength within it.

It was considered to be the stone of expansiveness which promoted the giving forth of the potential within and stimulated an inner glow in the person who wore it.

Topaz was thought also to induce a feeling of hope, like that which comes from watching the golden glow of sunrise as it marks the dawning of a new day and a new beginning.

Topaz was reputed to cause tension to flow away. In particular it was thought to absorb and disperse the negative vibrations of a troubled mind and was therefore considered to be a protection against depression and insomnia. One method of dispersing worries was to lie down with a topaz resting near the Third Eye chakra between and just above the eyebrows.

Topaz is a stone of encouragement for Brown Bears for it helps to dispel feelings of restriction and opens the mind to a recognition of new opportunities opening up before them. It stimulates both hope and joy within them and helps them to radiate these qualities to others.

6.10 POLARITY TOTEM: Wolf

Brown Bear people can be so self-reliant that they bear their own disappointments, griefs and sorrows in isolation and sometimes to the point where their own energy system can become blocked and they feel thwarted and despondent. They can find help by looking to their balancing totem, Wolf, and learning to rise above the material attachments of day-to-day practicalities by seeking the higher view that a more spiritual perspective can give them.

Like Brown Bears, Wolves have a tendency to keep themselves to themselves and like to withdraw from the world into their own clearly marked territory, but they are swift runners and have a capacity to climb the 'highest mountain'.

Bear people may need to recognize that the climbing they may need to do is of the mind and the spirit, and that which they may need to hunt is spirit development rather than the acquisition of material possessions alone. Their 'close-to-the-ground' practicality needs to be balanced with Wolf's spiritual far-sightedness.

6.11 PERSONALITY EXPRESSION
Adult

Hardworking, practical, eager, careful, plodding Brown Bear finds it difficult to let up from a round of constant activity.

Brown Bears have an eye for detail but easily lose sight of the main issue. Indeed, they can be quite perplexed when confronted with a problem, and have to break it down into smaller parts which can then be tackled one at a time.

It is the little things in life, and often issues which some other people might regard as relatively unimportant, which cause Brown Bears much anxiety. Sometimes this may be because Brown Bears find they cannot express themselves as clearly as they would like and this causes them problems, particularly in emotional relationships.

Brown Bears often find themselves on the receiving end of orders and of running about in the service of others. Since they are concerned about how other people regard them and are so considerate of others, they often allow themselves to be put into situations where advantage is taken of their warm-heartedness and generous nature.

On the one hand, Brown Bear are thoroughly dependable, working hard and long, and often taking on more than they can safely manage in their desire to fulfil other people's expectations. On the other hand, they

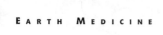

can reach a stage where they no longer want to do a particular task and pretend to be ill or make some other excuse rather than attempt to resolve the issue through discussion and negotiation.

Brown Bears tend to minimize their own talents and ignore their potentialities, sometimes because they allow their own active minds to create so many possibilities that they lose sight of the original idea before they can even begin to develop it.

Brown Bear people are creatures of habit, and it is not just a matter of schedules or the routine of storing things away in a particular place. They will even prefer to holiday in the same place because it has become familiar to them and they know their way around.

They are good-natured and show a surprising reasonableness over whatever is demanded of them, and make valuable friends. Brown Bears are essentially 'helpers', and are seemingly content to be in subordinate positions rather than in giving orders to others, though they generally prefer to be self-employed or to work on their own rather than alongside others whom they might find objectionable.

Positive traits: Discriminating. Meticulous. Analytical. Modest. Painstaking.

Negative traits: Fussy. Hypocritical. Finick. Fastidious.

Vocational possibilities: Art. Accounts. Bookkeeping. Journalism. Law. Medicine. Publishing work. Mechanics. Politics. Television. Radio. Stenography.

Child

The Brown Bear infant is generally more contented than most babies – what some people might describe as a 'good baby'. In their childhood they are easy to handle and seldom troublesome.

The Brown Bear child has a gentle disposition. It likes routine and orderliness because they provide a sense of security which is necessary to its well-being. Disorganization, confusion in the home or lack of clear authority at school can so disorientate the Brown Bear child as to cause not only anxiety but illness. The Brown Bear just needs to know where it stands.

Parent

Brown Bears usually make responsible and conscientious parents. The Brown Bear mother can be fussy with her children over neatness and tidiness and she can get upset if they come home dirty or tread mud over her clean floors. But though firm, she has a tenderness that usually elicits a willing response from her children.

Brown Bear fathers taken their parenthood seriously, too. They will make sacrifices in time as well as money in order to encourage and help their offspring with studies and with hobbies and sporting interests.

6.12 ROMANCE AND SEX

Because Brown Bears don't find it easy to express their deepest emotions, and hide their true feelings under a cloak of apparent casualness, they are often misunderstood. They are often embarrassed by the tide of feelings that well up inside them and in trying to overcome them they may appear aloof and even cold. So it usually takes time for Brown Bears to establish lasting relationships, but once they do find their true love their devotion and loyalty will never falter.

Brown Bears are gentle and tender lovers, taking their love-making slowly and considerately.

They have a strongly moralistic attitude, and though marriage and family are important to their sense of security and to their own psychological stability, they are likely to seek separation or divorce if their partner kicks over the traces once too often.

Compatibilities: Brown Bears are compatible with Goose and Beaver (those born between 22 December and 19 January and between 20 April and 20 May).

Spiritual sexuality: (–) The basic spiritual sexuality of Brown Bear is feminine, which indicates that they are inclined to be introverted, receptive and nurturing.

6.13 HEALTH

Stomach upsets, problems with the bowels, and skin eruptions suffered by Brown Bear people are likely to be the physical effects of inhibitions and limitations which they impose upon themselves, often through an abnormal concern over small and comparatively unimportant details which they allow to grow into big issues.

Mental upsets are likely to manifest in the stomach so Brown Bear are prone to stomach ulcers and colitis. The hands and feet are vulnerable areas also, particularly to injury.

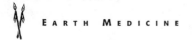

6.14 AFFINITY COLOUR: Brown and violet

Brown is the colour of the soil and of rocks and therefore of substance, so
people of this colour will have a materialistic attitude to life. It suggests
toil and effort and productivity, so people associated with this colour are
generally conscientious, hardworking and reliable, and show a certain
stamina in their undertakings.

Brown indicates a need for physical security and for 'belonging'. A
harmonious home or a den of one's own to which they can withdraw and
feel safe and comfortable is essential for Brown Bears.

In its lighter hues, brown indicates warmth and a desire to help others
less fortunate and especially the underdogs, or to undertake jobs that
others are reluctant to do. In its darker hues it indicates inflexibility,
inertia, obstinacy and a closed mind.

Like green, brown is a ray of balance. It is an 'earthing' colour whose
emphasis is on practical qualities.

Brown Bears are also influenced by violet, a colour at the spiritually
orientated end of the spectrum which helps to link the physical with the
non-physical, the objective with the subjective. It is a colour that augments
the spiritual aspects of the individual to correct imbalance that can result
from overemphasis on the purely physical aspects of living.

Violet is the colour of the sensitive – of the person quickly affected by
the moods of others and by the atmosphere of one's surroundings and
whose need is to take time to ponder and reflect before being committed to
a line of action initiated by another, or before pulling out of an environment in which one feels trapped or restricted.

Violet is also a colour associated with enchantment and fantasy. It is
when Brown Bears begin to fantasize or seek an escape from practical
reality by living in a nebulous dream world, that they need to seek the
balance that brown, at the more 'physical' end of the spectrum can provide
them with.

6.15 ADVANTAGEOUS TIMES

Best months of the year for Brown Bears are from 22 August to 21
September, 22 December to 19 January, and 20 April to 20 June.
Best day of the week is Wednesday.
Best times of the day are from 1 p.m. to 3 p.m.

6.16 OUTWARD (CONSCIOUS) AIM AND INNER (SUBCONSCIOUS) DESIRE

Brown Bear's conscious aim of striving for the best ways of dealing with physical and practical things is, in fact, an expression of a subconscious desire to locate the seed of spirituality that lies hidden in matter. This sifting through the experience of day-to-day practicalities is a search for the perfection of an inner reality wherein lies true security.

6.17 SPIRITUAL ALCHEMY

In Brown Bear, Earth is the force expressing itself through the form of work and service and Water is the force that causes flow from one experience to another, sensitive to the sentiments and feelings of others and drawing value from them. The emphasis is on the need for balance, for as Earth needs water for fertilization, so Water needs Earth to be of use. But they must be in balance. Too much Earth will lead to dryness and unfeeling, too much Water and Earth turns to mud and is unstable. In balance there is growth and fruitfulness and joy.

The directional influence is positive and hot moving to warm (+ +) and the elemental polarity is receptive with water (–) and Earth (–). The spiritual sexuality is feminine (–) so the personality leans more to passivity and receptivity. The combination is thus (+ +, – – and –).

6.18 Life-Challenges

Brown Bear people need to learn not to allow their desire for stability and dependence to become inflexibility and stubbornness, otherwise their growth and development will be hampered and they will find themselves caught on a cycle of repeating problems and difficulties.

Part of the purpose of some life-experiences is to demonstrate the need to balance the 'dream' with the practical realities of everyday life and by so doing learn to discriminate between what is true value and that which has served its purpose.

Must cultivate: Optimism. Tolerance. Lucidity.

Must avoid: Scepticism. Melancholy. Sloppiness. Nit-picking. Pettiness. Procrastination.

6.19 PRIMARY FUNCTION AND LIFE-PATH

The primary function of the Brown Bear is discrimination. Their life-path is one of processing what comes to them through life-experiences to discover what is of true value and to be retained and absorbed and ingested for future use, and what is superficial and can be eliminated.

But the path leads them beyond that innate ability to take things apart to see how they work. Its purpose is much more than that of satisfying curiosity. It is to discover the details that go into a creative idea so that they can be improved on and perfected.

Just as a tree puts down roots in order that it may have the capacity to form branches and thus explore the space around it, so Brown Bears tap the soil of their life-path in order to discover new ways of service and to extend their own sense of self.

At this stage of the journey on the Wheel of Life there awaits a realization that wisdom is not learned through struggle and conquest but only through the passage of time. It comes with the recognition that whatever is being searched for is to be found within the territory of one's own experience.

It is a path that leads to the acceptance of being content with what cannot be changed and to the exertion of energy only on those things that can. Wisdom comes through knowing the difference.

A prime purpose of this path is the acceptance that patience is a preliminary to solid achievement.

6.20 Tʜᴇ I Cʜɪɴɢ Tʀɪɢʀᴀᴍ: **Chen. The Arousing Thunder.**

Those born during the Harvesting Time are on the south-south-west direction on the Wheel of the Year.

The Arousing Thunder trigram represents expanding activity. It indicates growth that brings improvement. It suggests the arousal of creative potential and the liberation of ideas.

It emphasizes the importance of concentrating on a single, dominant idea or desire in bringing thoughts into manifestation and completion.

6.21 Hᴏᴡ ᴛᴏ Cᴏᴘᴇ ᴡɪᴛʜ Bʀᴏᴡɴ Bᴇᴀʀs

Appeal to the practical side of their nature. Show an interest in their work and concern for their welfare. Help them to see their ideas in terms of practical realities. Be logical.

Brown Bears don't like uncertainty and unpunctuality. So don't keep a Brown Bear waiting. They respond to genuine concern and affection and to gentleness. Get too emotional too quickly and Brown Bear is likely to turn and run.

Crow

SUMMARY

Birth dates:	22 September – 22 October (21 March – 19 April in the Southern hemisphere).
Earth influence:	The Falling Leaves Time.
Influencing wind:	The West Winds. *Totem*: Grizzly Bear.
Direction:	South-west.
Predominant elements:	Air with Earth.
Elemental clan:	Butterfly (Air) Clan. *Function*: Initiating ideas.
Birth and animal totem:	Crow.
Plant totem:	Ivy.
Mineral totem:	Azurite.
Polarity totem:	Falcon.
Affinity colour:	Blue.
Personality:	Charming. Friendly. Good-natured. Tolerant.
Feelings:	Sensitive.
Intention:	Justice.
Nature:	Co-operative.
Positive traits:	Idealistic. Romantic. Diplomatic.
Negative traits:	Indecisive. Frivolous. Gullible. Resentful.
Sex-drive:	Strong.
Compatibilities:	Otter and Deer.
Conscious aim:	Partnership.
Subconscious desire:	Harmony and beauty.
Life-path:	Harmonization.
I Ching trigram:	☳ Chen. Thunder. Desire for achievement.
Spiritual alchemy:	Yang predominates.
Must cultivate:	Decisiveness. Constancy. Inspiration. Stability.
Must avoid: Indecision.	Uncertainty. Inconsistency.
Starting totems:	Crow. Grizzly Bear. Butterfly. Ivy. Azurite. Falcon.

7. Crow

7.1 BIRTH MONTH: 22 September – 22 October

7.2 EARTH INFLUENCE: The Falling Leaves Time

This is the first cycle influenced by the spirit of the West and is the time of autumn when everything in Nature slows and there is consolidation as the internal structures are strengthened in preparation for the season of sleep and renewal which lies just ahead.

It is the time when the trees shed their leaves and when animals move to their winter locations, or begin to store up body fat for their period of hibernation, and when birds migrate to warmer climes.

Introspection is a quality of this time and people whose birthdays are during this period are influenced to drawn upon their inner resources and to look within rather than outside themselves for the solutions they seek.

7.3 SOLAR INFLUENCES

The Autumn Equinox around 22 September is another point of balance in the solar cycle when day and night are again equally matched to mark a 'change of gear' in the natural scheme of things. But whereas Nature was poised to spring into action at the Spring Equinox, it now prepares for resting as the Sun's power wanes and the contractive phase of the yearly cycle begins to predominate.

Anciently, this was a time of thanksgiving and of contemplation – of gratitude for what has been gathered during the fruitful times and of contemplation as the Wheel of Life turns towards the seasons of external barrenness and one looks to the strength that comes through the nourishment from within that sustains us. The related Sun sign is Libra.

7.4 INFLUENCING WIND: West Winds
DIRECTION: South-west

The west winds of autumn come with strength and power, and in human terms are the winds of maturity for they have a more definite direction, like the middle years of human life, compared with the blustery winds of trial and error that are experienced in young adulthood.

They are the winds that turn one away from engrossment in purely physical activity to contemplate not so much what has been achieved but what has been learned from the experience.

The West Winds bring a clearer dense of direction and purpose –

a clarity of mind for knowing where one is going and the comforting assurance that there is a supporting power behind you.

The influencing power of the West is concerned with consolidation and introspection. It helps in turned the mind from the material to the more spiritual aspects of life, and to making use of what has been gathered from the efforts of past activities.

It is a power that strengthens the resolve to discover one's own inner strengths and weaknesses and to put them to the test. And it provides the courage to reach out and to explore hitherto unknown realms.

The West is associated with autumn and with dusk, both of which herald periods of renewal. It also reflects the quality of maturity, and represents the middle years of life.

The totem animal of the West is the black-furred *grizzly*, the strongest of the bears, which busies itself in the autumn in preparation for the hibernation of winter.

The Amerindian regarded the grizzly as inward-looking because it appeared to be thoughtful about its actions, and tribal stories related how the animal was not only able to look within its own heart but also within the hearts of others and thereby acquire understanding.

The grizzly is a powerful animal, and as a totem reflects the selflessness of idealism, the wisdom of introspection, and the strength that comes from the spirit.

7.5 INFLUENCING ELEMENTS: **Air with Earth**

Elemental Earth has great sustaining power for it is the element of constancy and dependability. People influenced strongly by Earth are loyal and dependable partners, friends and colleagues.

The power of elemental Earth brings about an inner persistence which drives the person to try, try and try again after however many attempts, and to pick themselves up off the floor of apparent defeat and to press on again until victory is in sight.

Falling Leaves Time people are also strongly influenced by elemental Air which expresses itself through them in personal activity and through the mind.

Air stimulates and is energizing and refreshing, but it needs freedom to circulate or it becomes stale and oppressive. Air is associated with mental activity and with communication, so people born during this month will have lively minds and express themselves through words and ideas and like to communicate with others. However, their earthy stability may sometimes draw them into situations where they feel trapped or restricted.

Just as the air in which we move and breathe can be calm and refreshing, or when moved to gale force can become angry and destructive, so people born in Falling Leaves Time have a capacity to bring peace and harmony to a situation and to co-ordinate activities, or if their temper is aroused can become uncontrolled and have a quite shattering effect on those around them.

7.6 Elemental Clan: Butterfly (Air) Clan

Falling Leaves Time people are born into the Butterfly Clan and the strong influence by elemental Air explains why they find themselves always active and on the move and constantly shifting their attitude towards things.

Butterfly Clan people are the organizers and bringers of new ideas, the enthusiastic communicators.

7.7 Birth and Animal Totem: Crow

There are world-wide more than a hundred species of crow, and these include the rook, raven, magpie, and jackdaw. The crow is a stocky, black-feathered bird with a powerful beak and strong legs. It is one of the most adaptable birds and acclimatizes itself to most habitats.

The crow is essentially a forager, feeding largely on the ground from grain, root crops, fruit, nuts, carrion, insects and small animals. Its strong legs enable it to move rapidly over the ground. Crows usually forage in pairs or in groups. In winter it gathers in flocks and shares communal roosts.

Although it is regarded as a nuisance by farmers, the Amerindians looked upon its scavenging as a balancing activity in Nature's scheme of things. The crow was also rated as a 'teacher' bird because of its intelligence and its ability to be comfortable whether in the sky or on the ground, and because its group or 'tribal' habits appeared to be almost human. Native peoples have used the crow as a symbolic link between humanity and the environment and regarded its every appearance as having some message for its observer.

The raven is the largest member of the crow family, and has a diamond-shaped tail and long, pointed wings which can span up to 120 cm (4 ft). It has a stout, heavy bill and shaggy throat feathers. It builds its nest from twigs and sticks high up at the top of tall trees or on ledges and will attack birds that intrude on its space.

Like their totem, Crow people are not loners. They feel insecure on their own and prefer the company of others, feeling safety and security in numbers. So they work best as one of a group rather than on their own, and are happiest within the security of an organization.

Indeed, they have a strong sense of loyalty to the group or organization to which they belong and will readily defend it from attack, whether in word or deed.

Like the crow, they are often wary and suspicious, possibly because of past hurts under similar circumstances, and they may even appear to lack courage because of a tendency to back away from any situation that spells danger.

In ancient times, the crow and the raven were often associated with magik, which in simplistic terms is not supernatural or supernormal but the bringing of creative thought into physical reality. Crow people may appear to have an above-average ability to turn their wants and desires into material realities. The raven was also regarded anciently as the guardian and protector of 'secret' things, and Crow people are usually good at guarding confidences and can usually be trusted to be discreet.

The crow is a bird that has mastered the art of balance by the use of its wings, and is sensitive to changes in the atmosphere. Crow people are, as it were, hovering at the point of balance between different directions – a point of almost perpetual neutrality. It is, perhaps, because of this tendency that they are often indecisive and slow to make up their minds , whether in choosing something new to wear or determining a course of action. They have a knack of appreciating the qualities and advantages of whatever choices confront them and their problem is in actually making the choice. Once they have made a decision, however, they will act on it with conviction.

7.8 PLANT TOTEM: Ivy

Ivy (*Hedera helix*) is a tenacious evergreen plant that spirals its way around a tree and thrives in the dark half of the year. Its dark-green leathery leaves have three to five lobes. It flowers from August to October with small, globe-shaped yellow-green clusters. Its fruit is small black berries which ripen in winter and provide food for hungry birds.

The plant was used medicinally with care since it is poisonous. It was, however, used in the preparation of a wash to soothe conditions of the skin.

Ivy was regarded as a token of rebirth and regeneration. In European folk traditions it was paired with holly (ivy being regarded as essentially female and holly as male) and its tenacious and clinging quality and its ability to remain evergreen were symbolic of the survival of the essence of life.

The plant is particularly significant for Crow people, indicating the need to be tenacious and to hang on, especially in times of adversity or great change.

Ivy was used symbolically to make an arch that linked death with rebirth – indicating that what appeared to be an end was but a new beginning.

7.9 MINERAL TOTEM: Azurite

Azurite is a copper carbonate which has a opaque blue metallic appearance. It is a stone with a gentle and peaceful vibration which makes it particularly helpful as a focal point for meditation. There is a beauty in what may appear to be imperfections in the stone, but perhaps they are teaching us that though things may not appear to be perfect there is a potential for perfection within them.

Like azurite, Crow people have a gentle side to their nature which enables them to harmonize situations in which they are involved.

Crow people should wear azurite for it will help them to connect more powerfully with Earth energies and obtain a clearer insight into their own natures. It can also help them to expand their awareness and to become more clear-sighted. It can be worn as a ring, preferably on the right hand, or just carried on the person.

7.10 POLARITY TOTEM: Falcon

Like their birth totem, Crow people are capable of soaring from one thing to another and from the security and satisfaction of material acquisitions to the elevation that can be derived from spiritual experiences. Their difficulty is inconsistency and an ambivalence which makes them wary and hesitant about making decisions, so to attain their personal balance they need the foresight, fearlessness, and driving energy of the Falcon.

Once Crows find their point of balance and learn to direct their energies effectively, they can be the most helpful of all people because they enjoy the satisfaction of sharing.

7.11 PERSONALITY EXPRESSION
Adult

Restless, good-natured, artistic, talkative Crow. Crows are people who enjoy new things and new experiences, but their restlessness is not the hustling and bustling kind. With them it is that once they have explored one avenue of interest or one relationship they are anxious to move on to the next.

They are generally pleasant and good-natured folk, but easily affected by atmosphere, either of a place or of that generated by a person or group of people, and if that is adverse to them they are likely to become sulky, moody and irritable.

Crow people show the two sides of their nature more readily than most. At times they are cheerful, gregarious and fun to be with. At other times they can be annoying, quarrelsome, stubborn and morose. Similarly, they may have periods when they put every ounce of energy into their work and give the impression of being workaholics, but when they do decide to take a break and relax, their reluctance to start work again may make them appear to be lethargic and even lazy. Crows do need to recharge their batteries from time to time, and once that's done they usually apply themselves enthusiastically again to their work and engage in another nose-to-the-grindstone phase.

Crows dislike muddle and confusion. They like things to be tidy and efficient whether it is at their place of work or in their home.

Easy-going individuals, Crows usually fit in well with groups of people, and their tact and diplomacy can help to mould a group together into a harmonious team. Crows are not loners. Indeed, they can become quite depressed working alone or left to their own devices. They 'come alive' in a group or with a partner. Crows just have to be able to share.

Crows dislike quarrels and contention and emotional upsets and their tendency to be all things to all men sometimes results in others accusing them of being 'two-faced'. By nature they make good negotiators.

Their desire for balance and justice is a reflection of their place on the Earth Web which marks the period of dusk in the daily cycle when Nature reaches a point of balance, and of autumn in the yearly cycle when day and night are of equal length. Just as there are turning-points in the natural cycle, so are Crows at a turning-point in the cycle of spiritual evolution, balanced between the material, physical world of that which can be seen and felt and experienced with the physical senses, and that of the realm of the invisible which can only be discerned with the spirit. So Crows, though practical and with their feet on the ground, have a deep interest in the mysteries of life.

Positive traits: Idealistic. Diplomatic. Romantic. Easy-going. Friendly. Co-operative.

Negative traits: Indecisive. Resentful. Frivolous. Gullible.

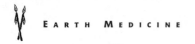

Vocational possibilities: Arts. Antiques. Aviation. Architecture.
Engineering. Mechanics. Military. Objets d'Art. Painting. Politics. Property.

Child

The Crow baby is usually the beautiful well-behaved infant that captures
the heart of whoever is around. As infants, Crows appear less prone to
throwing tantrums than most little ones and are usually contented and
well-mannered.

The Crow child shows a reluctance to make decisions at an early age.
It prefers not to be faced with choices, whether it is about what it is going
to eat or wear or play with. It does not require everything to be imposed
upon it, but it does need guidance in helping it to make choices. But it
simply won't be hurried into making up its mind.

This hesitancy may continue as the Crow child gets older and can be
mistaken for stubbornness when it is, in fact, cautiousness. Their desire is
to please, but if their hesitancy is handled clumsily it is a trait which can
develop into a fear of making mistakes or misjudgements.

Crow children are usually bright and inquisitive.

Parent

Crows don't usually rush into parenthood. They prefer to wait until they
have a home well-established before starting a family.

The male Crow makes a devoted father who exerts a quiet authority
over his offspring.

The Crow mother is caring and gentle, but firm when necessary. But
her children will always take second place to her partner.

7.12 ROMANCE AND SEX

Crows are romantics and so much in love with love that they are likely
to settle down with a partner before a true relationship has been firmly
established with the consequence that they may come to regret it later on.

They have their dreams of perfect love, but in the world of practical
reality discover that perfection is less easy to find and their search for the
perfect mate makes them appear to be fickle and flirtatious.

Male Crows can be charming, considerate and thoughtful, and say all
the right things that make a woman feel good. Crow women can be affectionate and seductive and have a soft femininity that attracts men, but
they rarely let their emotions rule their judgement in practical matters.

Sex is important to Crows, though it may be the invigoration of the chase and the stimulation of the preliminaries to sexual union that excites them more than the act itself. They usually make tender and gentle lovers and have a sexual appetite that some might regard as excessive.

Compatibilities: Crows are compatible with Otters and Deer (those born between 20 January and 18 February and between 21 May and 20 June).

Spiritual sexuality: (+) The basic spiritual sexuality of Crows is masculine, so they are energetic, extroverted, and initiating.

7.14 HEALTH

Over-indulgence is the biggest threat to the physical well-being of Crows. The organ most affected is likely to be the kidneys. Crows may have muscular problems, usually in the region of the lower back.

Exercise of the diaphragm and the area of the body around the waist is particularly beneficial to Crows for in the inner body it is that area which separates the upper and lower halves and might be described as the balancing-point of the body.

7.14 AFFINITY COLOUR: Blue

Blue searches beyond the practicalities of physical existence for it is the colour of the sky and explores the infinity of spirituality. Blue is also the colour of the oceans so those affected by it will strive to search the depths of profound wisdom and introspective awareness.

Blue suggests tranquillity and devotion as aspiration. The colour can be relaxing and soothing, but also stimulating and uplifting. So those affected by the blue ray will be adaptable and reflect its qualities too.

Blue symbolizes harmony and truth and represents spirituality and cosmic energy. It is a colour that raises the consciousness to spiritual levels and in the human aura indicates integrity, sincerity and compassion.

The blue ray brings to those born during the Falling Leaves Time a quietness of spirit that desires orderliness and freedom from contention. It is the colour that draws the consciousness to look inward for the true values.

Blue-affected people have a strong sense of duty and faithfulness. They are sensitive to the needs of others. They are sociable and caring.

Blue is the colour of peace, so blue-affected people are usually diplomatic and discreet. They are good 'fixers', able to bring opposing parties into compatible relationships. Like the colour, they are good mixers who are likeable and generally get on well with others.

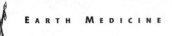

7.15 ADVANTAGEOUS TIMES

Best months of the year for Crow people are from 22 September to
22 October, 20 January to 18 February, and 20 April to 20 June.
Best day of the week is Friday.
Best times of the day are from 3 p.m. to 5 p.m.

7.16 OUTWARD (CONSCIOUS) AIM AND
INNER (SUBCONSCIOUS) DESIRE

Crows' outward aim is co-operation in the desire for harmony and beauty.

Crows are at the point in their spiritual evolution that can be likened to
the pause between heartbeats or where a pendulum pauses momentarily in
its swing. It is a state of static equilibrium between change – a point of
balance. The purpose of balance is to determine action. It is not inaction,
but the state from which arises a new cycle, another pulsation.

The inner desire is to find that moment of change, of decision, that
point of balance, when yin changes to yang. So part of the purpose of
Crow life-experiences is to put them into places of having to make
decisions that are wise judgements.

7.17 SPIRITUAL ALCHEMY

Crows are influenced by Air, which is the element of mind, and the force
that is constantly on the move and circulating, and by Earth, which is the
element of practical reality.

Too much Air and Crow is living in an airy-fairy world of ideas and
dreams which exist only in the mind. Too much Earth and Crow becomes
bogged down, limited and restricted. Crow has to balance the two, then
the ideas and dreams generated under the Air influence are brought down
to Earth and into physical manifestation.

The directional influence is warm moving to cool (+ –), the elemental
polarities are Earth (–) and Air (+), and the spiritual sexuality is masculine
(+) emphasizing the personality towards action and outgoing concern.

7.18 LIFE-CHALLENGES

Crows find themselves in situations where there is a dependence on others
and a need for consensus, but the real lesson from a repetition of these
experiences is the learning to make one's own decisions and to take
personal responsibility for one's own life. It is acquiring the capacity to
co-operate with others and to share without losing one's individuality and
independence.

Must cultivate: Decisiveness. Constancy. Impartiality. Gracefulness. Inspiration. Artistic nature.

Must avoid: Indecision. Dependence on others. Deceitfulness. Inconsistency.

7.19 PRIMARY FUNCTION AND LIFE-PATH

The primary function of Crow is harmonization through bringing together. Put another way, it is the discovery of new beginnings through the harmony of sharing.

A dictionary definition of harmony is the bringing together of different notes or surfaces or objects to form an orderly and agreeable whole.

Through the experience of developing an ability to see things from the perspective of others and cultivating a capacity to integrate seemingly opposite points of view, Crows are presented with the opportunity of bringing about a variety of agreeable partnerships which are able to operate on a different level of activity. In this way their own spiritual evolution is being carried to a higher or more sensitive level.

Their life-path leads them to a recognition of the necessity for the utmost integrity in decisions and actions because every action creates an equivalent reaction which rebounds to form a karmic pattern for the future. It is the High Self which requires and demands justice, and every decision and action brings ultimately its equivalent compensation.

The prime purpose for those on this path is to be able to discern between principles and passions.

7.20 THE I CHING TRIGRAM: Chen. The Arousing Thunder.

▬▬ ▬▬ Those born in the Falling Leaves Time are on the south-west direction
▬▬▬▬ on the Wheel of the Year.

The appearance of this trigram, with its two broken lines at the top and a solid line at the bottom is sometimes likened to a cup, and a cup suggests receptivity. It suggests a receptacle for ideas which can be mixed together to form a harmonious whole.

The Chen trigram indicates the arousal into activity which, like thunder, heralds the bringing about of change which is in accordance with the harmonious natural order and rhythms. In essence, it is the desire for achievement.

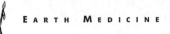

7.21 HOW TO COPE WITH CROWS

Don't mistake Crow's friendliness for affection. Keep to the point in your conversation. Crows like to have things explained to them clearly and logically, and dislike long-winded wafflers almost as much as fast-talking, high-pressure salesmen. Don't get involved in coarse conversation with a group that includes Crow. Crows are offended by vulgarity, though they are often too diplomatic to reveal their feelings.

Snake

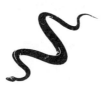

SUMMARY

Birth dates:	23 October – 22 November (20 April – 20 May in the Southern hemisphere).
Earth influence:	The Frost Time.
Influencing wind:	The West Winds. *Totem:* Grizzly Bear.
Direction:	West.
Predominant elements:	Water with Earth.
Elemental clan:	Frog (Water) Clan. *Function:* mental involvement.
Birth and animal totem:	Snake.
Plant totem:	Thistle.
Mineral totem:	Amethyst.
Polarity totem:	Beaver.
Affinity colour:	Violet.
Personality:	Intense. Impulsive. Ambitious. Determined. Mysterious.
Feelings:	Hidden.
Intention:	Introspection.
Nature:	Inquiring.
Positive traits:	Purposeful. Discerning. Imaginative.
Negative traits:	Resentful. Stubborn. Secretive. Suspicious.
Sex-drive:	Intense.
Compatibilities:	Woodpeckers and Wolves.
Conscious aim:	Satisfaction.
Subconscious desire:	Spiritual union.
Life-path:	Sensitivity.
I Ching trigram:	☷ K'un. The Receptive Earth. Natural response.
Spiritual alchemy:	Yin predominates.
Must cultivate:	Determination. Adaptability. Creativity.
Must avoid:	Egotism. Arrogance. Envy. Despondency.
Starting totems:	Snake. Grizzly bear. Frog. Thistle. Amethyst. Beaver.

8. Snake

8.1 BIRTH MONTH: 23 October – 22 November

8.2 EARTH INFLUENCE: The Frost Time

People born in the Frost Time abound with ideas and enthusiasm, but when they allow their energies to run away with them uncontrolled, they often find their schemes 'frozen' to a standstill by the frosty reception of the outside world. They need to apply the warmth of emotion to cold intellect to keep such energies flowing.

Conversely, they need also to learn that it is sometimes wiser to put an idea into 'deep freeze' until the climate is right. Learning the art of timing is one of the greatest lessons of experience to be learned by people born in this Time, for although they have sound ideas and good intentions, they all too often find frustration because they have launched out at an inappropriate time. Their impatience in 'running ahead of themselves' is, perhaps, their greatest handicap.

8.3 SOLAR INFLUENCES

Those born at this Time are associated with the setting Sun and with the season of autumn, and with the years of maturity in human life. They are aligned with the powers of twilight which change the face of the Earth and motivate them towards the freedom of idealism. They have an inquisitiveness of spirit that drives them on to uncover purpose in existence and this quest to discover the mysteries of life is true maturity.

Nature at this time of the year helps us to understand the principle of transformation and regeneration which has such a strong influence on those born at this time, for although autumn is the season of defoliation when the trees become barren, the fallen leaves which have been discarded will decompose to provide nutrients for the Earth beneath and nourishment for the future development of the trees from which they came. Frost is a reminder of the death which winter represents. It changes to water when warmed but is renewed overnight.

A pivotal point of the entire yearly cycle is located in this period. Anciently it was recognized as the time when the year ended and a new yearly cycle began. This 'twilight' period had significance in another way among ancient peoples for it was seen, too, as the space between two realms – between the visible world of physical manifestation and the unseen realm of the spirit.

It was celebrated as a festival among pagan peoples on the eve of
1 November. The ancient Celts called is Samhain, which meant 'Summers'
End', but the celebrations continued merrily throughout the first week of
November. Blazing ritual bonfires symbolized the burning of all the worries
and problems accrued during the past year and these were the true origin
of Bonfire Night in Britain on 5 November and had far greater significance
than the memorial of Guy Fawkes' plot to blow up the Houses of
Parliament. It was a time for getting rid of weaknesses and the things
which had served their purpose but were no longer relevant – of shedding
what had gone before so that renewal became possible and effective. The
fires were also used to cook the meat of animals which could not be kept
over Winter. The result of the year's work was seen.

Just as twilight is an 'in-between' period separating daytime from
night, and autumn comes in between summer and winter, so Samhain was
looked upon as a time when the visible and invisible realms 'overlapped'.
So it was a time to remember those who had died and had departed the
Earth life, and when the movement of the Earth tides had brought the
physical and the spiritual closer together, and when this closeness to
departed loved ones could be more keenly felt.

The Christian Church attempted to kill off the old festival by making
1 November All Saints Day, Samhain Eve on 31 October becoming All
Souls Day, All Hallows Eve or Hallowe'en. The original festival was
denigrated by associating it with demons and witches, and ghosts and
goblins. In modern times, Hallowe'en has become popularized, particularly
in the United States, as a time for rather weird fun, for dressing up in
costumes and masks, and of pumpkin and turnip lanterns, and an occasion
for 'trick or treat' suggesting the trickiness of little 'demons' and the need
to placate them, all of which is a distortion of the true significance of this
ancient festival.

The related sign in Sun astrology for those born at this Time is Scorpio.

8.4 INFLUENCING WIND: West Winds
DIRECTION: West

The west winds bring their influence of adaptability to those born in the
Frost Time and enable them to feel comfortable, whether they are handling
the material things of the Earth or considering the spiritual principles of
the 'Sky', and urges them to pass on their knowledge of these realms to
others.

The west winds bring power and strength, but since the West is the direction of introspection and selflessness, it is a power that stems from within rather than from without, and has a probing intensity that uncovers what has been hidden. Its strength is that which it gives to emotional endurance.

The totem of the West is the *grizzly bear*, which combines strength with gentleness – two apparently opposite yet complementary qualities which become increasingly evident in the more developed people of this time (see section 7.4).

8.5 INFLUENCING ELEMENTS: **Water with Earth**

Elemental Earth provides the nourishing power for things to appear and the dispersing energy for things to disappear again, and although Earth is the substance that provides stability and solidity, it is also the influence of transformation. It is this aspect of transformation that is of particular relevance to people born in the Frost Time for their whole lives are concerned primarily with change and renewal.

Endurance, resourcefulness and perseverance are qualities associated with elemental Earth.

The influence of elemental Water is associated with fluidity, flexibility, and adaptability – qualities which people born at this time also find themselves having to acquire.

8.6 ELEMENTAL CLAN: **The Frog (Water) Clan**

People born during the Frost Time are of the Frog Clan and closely involved with elemental Water. The fluidity of their nature causes them to be easily carried away in their thirst for new ideas and fresh experiences. They have an ability to bring renewal and freshness to any project in which they become involved, but rarely stay with it long enough to reap the full reward for all their efforts, preferring to 'swim' off in their quest for another new experience.

Frog Clan people are able to tap into the flow of creative and healing energies and to carry them into areas of need. Though they can be practical and 'earthy' and enjoy the feeling of material things around them, they are rarely satisfied for long and seem more at home in exploring the intangible things of life.

8.7 BIRTH AND ANIMAL TOTEM: **Snake**

Although the snake is a reptile that is looked upon with a certain abhorrence and repugnance in some cultures, and frequently among Caucasians feared and hated, Native peoples treat it with respect and, indeed, regard it as possessing many special powers. In particular, the snake represents the power of transformation and renewal through its ability to shed its skin frequently.

The snake is a limbless creature which is able to glide along by the forward and backward movement of its system of belly scales, which are called scutes. It has expandable jaws, and teeth which slope inward and towards the back of its mouth. It eats rats, mice, lizards and frogs, and also likes insects.

Its forked tongue is a sensing device for both taste and smell, and it is highly sensitive to vibrations. The snake sheds its skin periodically, leaving behind a tissue-like impression of its body and scales.

Like the snake, people born in the Frost Time are inclined to make dramatic changes in their lives, frequently shedding past attachments and ties, and appearing to start anew.

Snake people make these changes for the best possible reasons, but sometimes at inopportune times, thus bringing unnecessary trauma and suffering upon themselves. An important purpose in their lives is learning the art of timing. As change doesn't always come easily to them, Snake people do adapt themselves to any new situation and endeavour to make the best of it.

As snakes have a keen sense of sight and are able to fix their prey with a hypnotic-like stare that freezes it to the spot, so Snake people have a tendency to look you straight in the eye with a stare that seems to penetrate right through to the soul, and some people find this experience unsettling and even disturbing. It is as if the Snake person can see right into the secrets of your very being.

Native peoples knew the snake as a creature that is slow to anger, so it was considered symbolic of the quality of tolerance. Indeed, the purpose of many experiences encountered by Snake people in their lives is to enable them to learn the virtues of patience and tolerance.

In ancient times the snake was a protector of the Mystery Schools, guarding access to knowledge and wisdom from those whose motives might be questionable. The snake is also the protector of hallucinatory plants and Snake people can be especially helpful to those who suffer from alcohol or drug abuse.

The Snake who turned into a flying serpent was a symbol of a god among the ancient Mayan Indians. This is not implying that Snake people are turning into 'gods', but many of them are aware of aspirations that thrust them onwards and upwards, however adverse the situation, and this is intrinsic within the nature they may have taken on for this lifetime and an indication that they are involved in a lifelong process of transformation. It is a transformation of purely selfish purposes, of benefit only to the individual, into constructive energies that can be shared by others. It is the abandonment of the ability to wound and its replacement with the power to heal and to bring enlightenment and hope.

In Hinduism the god Shiva symbolizes a similar principle in the legendary story in which the coiled snake turns into a garland of flowers and covers him in beauty.

8.8 PLANT TOTEM: Thistle

Thistles have thick, prickly leaves and dense flower-heads with purple flowers. Thistle have a thick, fibrous stem and grow usually in clumps of varying heights of 30–180 cm (1–6 ft).

Modern man regards the thistle as a nuisance, but to the Amerindian it had good and wholesome qualities. It was used to cure most aches and pains, and was particularly effective in dealing with digestive disorders. It was also considered useful against all kinds of poisons.

Like the thistle with its prickles, Snake people have a 'mechanism' that prevents people from getting too close to them and really understanding what makes them tick. As a result, Snake people are often misunderstood and their true worth underrated. This need to keep people at bay is because of a feeling of vulnerability.

One of the lessons Snake people need to learn from life experiences is the need for a strong root in the Earth – like the thistle – for only then can their abundant energies be channelled fruitfully. Like the thistle, their growth depends upon how well they cultivate their talents and ability.

The thistle is rich in vitamins. The American Indians peeled the root and ate it raw, and the seeds were often eaten raw or roasted. The leaves were dried and used as a herbal tea.

8.9 MINERAL TOTEM: Amethyst

The amethyst is a crystalline quartz which is transparent and coloured light or dark violet or purple. Its colour is due to its manganese and iron thio-cyanate content and its power is due in part to its titanium content.

Titanium is a metallic element which has an 'upward striving' quality and it is perhaps not without significance that it is used in certain alloys in the construction of space rockets. The word titanium is derived from 'Titan', the mythological giant with great strength and power who strove to break free from the Underworld. So the amethyst is an aid to those 'upward striving' aspirations which develop spiritual unfoldment and creative thinking. It is reputed to have an ability to support its wearer in dealings with those in positions of power and authority or influence – in other words, with people in high places.

In ancient times the amethyst was considered to be a protection against intoxication, but this was not the intoxication of strong drink, but rather the manipulative or persuasive powers of fascination of those who sought control over people. The amethyst was used as a protective device because it puts an auric skin around its wearer and acts like a shield in warding off any attempt by another person to appropriate one's power.

The amethyst has an energy pattern that makes it a suitable aid to meditation and opens up the inner sight (the insight) and imparts spiritual power, and it is from this ancient knowledge that the amethyst was given religious significance and is used on the rings of bishops. This energy pattern has a calming effect on the emotions and helps to balance the energies of the physical plane with those on more subtle levels, so a person who is emotionally vulnerable may find that the stone has a harmonizing effect and they are not so easily carried away by their emotions.

In northern Europe there are 'old wives' tales' about the amethyst being a protection against storms and lightning. One Medicine Man told me that the Indian, who was so used to the open-air life, recognized that lightning never struck the wearer of an amethyst.

The energy pattern of the amethyst acts like a filter to absorb and repel vibrations which are not beneficial to the wearer and amplifies those rays that are; thus it can be used as a centre of focus. It does not operate through a particular chakra but works directly through that part of the energy body in the area in which it is worn or held.

The amethyst is thus symbolic of courage and of transformation, and Snake people can reflect something of its qualities, particularly in adverse situations, though the amethyst harmonizes with all.

8.10 POLARITY TOTEM: Beaver

Snake people are generally reluctant to reveal to others, even to their loved ones, their innermost feelings and the secrets of the heart, and because of this they are thought to be secretive and somewhat mysterious. They give the appearance of casting aside old beliefs and ideas with great ease, and seem able to put the past behind them with apparent unconcern. Indeed they involve themselves completely in any new situation. None the less, they are not as malleable as they may seem and, indeed, change often causes them much inner suffering. Their intensity and seriousness of purpose is their strength, but is also their weakness.

Beavers can help Snakes to find their point of balance, for they demonstrate the quality of patient endurance and a stability which Snake people need. They also have a sense of fun, and it is this quality which Snakes particularly need to put them in balance. Snakes have to learn not to take life so seriously.

8.11 Personality Expression
Adult

Mysterious, sensuous, ambitious, impulsive Snake is a deep, intense and determined person.

Snakes are people of extremes: they can reach the heights of material, mental or spiritual affairs, but they also plumb the depths. They are prone to dropping quickly and suddenly into the pit of gloom and despair, only to pick themselves up, dust themselves down, and start climbing back upwards once again. Snakes are never 'finished' for they make the most surprising comebacks. Regeneration is the name of their game.

They have magnetic personalities which can be quite devastating to some people. Their piercing eyes and hypnotic gaze can be penetrating and unsettling.

Snakes have deep feelings but manage to hid their emotions behind a cool exterior which is typical of their protective and secretive nature. They are a fascinating mixture of opposites. They can be childishly naive or penetratingly critical, impulsive or rational, enthusiastic or lethargic, tolerant or bigoted, spiritually minded or materialistic. Whatever it is, they do nothing by halves. They have an intensity which makes them prone to sudden attachments – and equally sudden detachments. They have good analytical powers that enable them to make sound judgements with objective impartiality – a quality which enables them to act in clear and decisive ways.

Like their totem, Snake people move slowly and carefully on smooth ground, but more speedily when the going is tough. Snakes make the most progress when there are obstacles in the way, for they respond to challenges.

Snake people are generous, not only with their money but with their time too. They like to surround themselves with luxury and are likely to be self-indulgent at times and go to excesses in food, drink and sex.

Positive traits: Purposeful. Determined. Discerning. Powerful. Imaginative.

Negative traits: Jealous. Resentful. Stubborn. Obstinate. Secretive. Suspicious. Intractable.

Vocational possibilities: Arts. Detection. Exploration. Law. Policing. Military. Politics. Transport. Scientific research. Medicine. Surgery.

Child

Snakes are usually strong and active babies, and their sense of curiosity soon displays itself. Snake infants are into everything, and there comes a time when even a playpen won't restrict them. They will find ways of being up and out of them.

The Snake child can be quite a challenge, even to the most competent parent, and can display revengeful anger towards other children who step on its toys. But Snake children are quick learners and their penetrating minds and sharp intellect can make them among the leaders of their class.

Parent

Snakes make good parents. Father Snake will teach his children respect and a sense of responsibility and won't let them run riot. Indeed, he can be rather stern and sometimes quite forbidding. His efforts in teaching his children what life is about may not be appreciated until later – perhaps not until his children have kids of their own – and then they may be grateful for the fatherly guidance they have had.

The Snake woman makes a devoted mother whose offspring will always feel secure under her watchful eye. She will provide motherly support and encouragement in all their endeavours and be sympathetic and helpful in times of difficulty. As they get older she becomes a wise counsellor and friend.

8.12 ROMANCE AND SEX

Snakes need a constant show of affection. They have to be loved in order to show love, then they are likely to make love with fierce abandon.

Snakes make loyal and supportive partners, putting their mate's happiness right at the top of their list of priorities, and they will demonstrate this in many practical and pleasing ways.

Snake men are considerate and understanding to the woman who understands them, but they can be domineering and obstructive with an unsuitable partner.

Snake women are strongly individualistic. Confident and self-assured, they can be domineering and overbearing. The female Snake has a sharp tongue and can be brutally frank with it. She will always insist on having the last word.

The homes of Snake people are usually comfortable and tastefully decorated and furnished, but they will not flinch about uprooting and moving to an unfamiliar location and start a new home all over again.

Snakes have a highly developed sex-drive which can be obsessive. Their love-making can be passionate and even wild. But again, it's total sex or none at all!

Compatibilities: Snake people are compatible with Wolves and Woodpeckers (those born between 19 February and 20 March, and 21 June and 21 July).

8.13 HEALTH

Snake's ice-cool temperament is likely to freeze up the emotions and together with a bottling up of energies caused by stress, can result in nervous disorders, stomach ulcers, and intestinal complaints like constipation.

Snake's frigid emotional nature is often compensated for by a heightened flow of sexual and menstrual fluids and these produce an abundance of sexual energy which if denied physical or creative outlets may cause problems in the reproductive system.

8.14 AFFINITY COLOUR: Violet

Snake people are influenced by the violet ray. Since antiquity, violet has been associated with religious devotion or spiritual values, with magik and mysticism, and with glamour and richness. Violet is a mixture of red and blue. Red, as we have already seen, shows energy and vitality, while blue indicates compassion and kindliness. Violet embraces all of these principles.

Purple is a rather heavier and more solemn colour and expresses feelings of grandeur. In an aura it indicates clairvoyance but it can also indicate eccentricity and pride that expresses itself in pomposity.

Violet in an aura is the colour of the mystic, but also the positive assurance that lacks dogmatism.

Snake people need the soothing rays of violet for it helps to restore their inner balance and to calm the mind and body, especially in times of stress or periods of despondency.

Violet brings with it peacefulness and tranquillity and its influence is towards involvement which makes no demands or attachments and thus arouses no anxieties.

8.15 ADVANTAGEOUS TIMES
Best months of the year for Snake people are from 23 October to 22 November, 19 February to 19 April, and 21 June to 21 July.
Best day of the week is Tuesday.
Best times of the day are from 5 a.m. to 7 a.m. and 5 p.m. to 7 p.m.

8.16 OUTWARD (CONSCIOUS) AIM AND INNER (SUBCONSCIOUS) DESIRE
The conscious aim of Snake people is to satisfy their impetuous desires which experience ultimately teaches them produces their most persistent problems and anxieties. So this aim leads to a realization that personal desire needs to be not only controlled but changed and elevated and that this can be achieved only by a letting go.

The inner desire is for union with the immortal self which will bring about an expansion of consciousness but which requires the elimination of those things that are no longer necessary to growth and reconstruction, so personal sacrifice is needed to find the deeper meaning of life.

The urge to penetrate into what exists around them in their circle of awareness stems from the desire to find ways of extending awareness through transition from one level of experience to another and thus to further their own self-development. But this activity requires sacrifice. As the snake sacrifices the skin that has held it together in the past, so the Snake person is required to cast off that which they have regarded as essential for past growth but now holds them locked in and constrained from further development.

8.17 SPIRITUAL ALCHEMY
As Earth needs Water for the fertilization of what it needs to produce, so Water needs Earth to hold it so that it can be used.

Snake, and its complementary opposite Beaver are on the Earth–Fire horizontal axis of the equal-armed cross within the Earth Medicine Wheel, with Salmon and Otter (Water and Air) on the vertical axis. Each of these four personality 'groups' is characterized by determination and strength of purpose.

Snake is strongly influenced by Earth and Water, but polarized by Fire and balanced by Air, indicating that strength of will and determination is needed to lift the self from the clinging attractions of Earth and up through the waters of emotion and transmuting fire into the Air of detachment which is soul purposefulness.

8.18 LIFE-CHALLENGES

Snake people are presented in their lives with what seem to be immense tasks to overcome, and it may even appear that they themselves have brought about the very circumstances that are so threatening.

My mentors have told me that what is happening is that the collective limiting factors of past errors which may even have developed over several lifetimes, are being brought to the surface for elimination in the present Snake incarnation. These challenges arise from inner unconscious levels and confront the individual with what appear to be formidable tasks involving sudden and dramatic change.

To the Amerindian, change was synonymous with death, for change was the death of what had gone before and the birth of what was to become. So the tests and trials and crises encountered frequently by Snake people are their points of reorientation – the facing up to what has held back the physical, emotional and mental nature to prevent the evolution of the soul, so that these can at last be overcome to enable regeneration on another level.

In some cultures the equivalent of the Snake was the scorpion – a creature that hides in the darkness and stings and wounds. The scorpion was symbolic of the unevolved elements of the 'lower' self which I have just mentioned.

Must cultivate: Determination. Resourcefulness. Agility. Flexibility. Adaptability. Creativity.

Must avoid: Egotism. Obstinacy. Arrogance. Suspicion. Jealousy. Envy. Despondency.

8.19 PRIMARY FUNCTION AND LIFE-PATH

The primary function of Snake is to expand the range of awareness through elimination of that which has served its purpose and is no longer needed and to attain union with the immortal self through renewal.

Sensitivity is the path of Snake and its purpose is to enable the vital life-forces to be recognized and made use of for further progress and spiritual evolution. Latent abilities and intuitive and creative skills leading to true fulfilment develop once self-discipline and emotional stability have been established.

It is a path that leads to a recognition that it is necessary to sacrifice something of value in order to attain that which is of much greater worth. Its emphasis is on the relinquishing of one thing in order for something better to emerge, and the need to be willing to trust the unseen workings of the unconscious to bring about a better life.

A prime purpose for being on this path is to attain the willingness to adapt.

8.20 THE I CHING TRIGRAM: K'un. The Receptive Earth.

▬ ▬ Those born during the Frost Time are on the West direction of the
▬ ▬ Wheel of the Year.

The receptive Earth is the nourishing womb. It is also symbolic of the subconscious mind. It indicates that aggressive attempts to attain what is desired by forceful means will lead to confusion and instability. Success comes through quiet cultivation and persistence and through responding naturally. The responsive quality of Nature reveals that what is contained within must come forth, but only in accordance with natural laws. The seed must first root itself, then put forth shoots and come into leaf before it can burst into blossom and eventually bear fruit. This is the lesson Snake must learn.

8.21 HOW TO COPE WITH SNAKES

Be straightforward. Snakes dislike deviousness. Be precise. Snakes get bored with long explanations. Be true your world. Snakes won't hang around it they think you cannot be trusted.

Don't arouse their anger. Snakes have short memories, but they never forget a hurt.

Owl

Summary

Birth dates:	23 November – 21 December (21 May – 20 June in the Southern hemisphere).
Earth influence:	The Long Nights Time.
Influencing wind:	The West Winds. *Totem*: Grizzly Bear.
Direction:	North-west.
Predominant elements:	Fire with Earth.
Elemental clan:	Hawk (Fire) Clan. *Function*: changing things.
Birth and animal totem:	Owl.
Plant totem:	Mistletoe.
Mineral totem:	Obsidian.
Polarity totem:	Deer.
Affinity colour:	Gold.
Personality:	Jovial. Warm-hearted. Adventurous. Independent.
Feelings:	Warm.
Intention:	Objectivity.
Nature:	Sincere.
Positive traits:	Versatile. Adaptable. Scrupulous.
Negative traits:	Restless. Tactless. Boisterous.
Sex-drive:	Adventurous.
Compatibilities:	Falcons and Salmon.
Conscious aim:	Understanding.
Subconscious desire:	Determination.
Life-path:	Elevation.
I Ching trigram:	☶ Ken. The Still Mountain. The need for singleness of purpose.
Must cultivate:	Concentration. Optimism. Enthusiasm.
Must avoid:	Over-indulgence. Exaggeration. Greed.
Spiritual alchemy:	Yang and yin balanced.
Starting totems:	Owl. Grizzly bear. Hawk. Mistletoe. Obsidian. Deer.

9. Owl

9.1 BIRTH MONTH: 23 November – 21 December

9.2 EARTH INFLUENCE: The Long Nights Time

Those born in the Long Nights Time are thoughtful people with an ability to seek out things from the minds of others as well as from within themselves.

This is the last of the cycles influenced by the spirit of the West with its qualities of introspection, and is the time of new opportunities.

At this time of the year in the Northern hemisphere, the air is crisp and clean and one can see clearly in all directions, and to people born at this time, growth is a question of determining the direction of one's life and of having a clear 'sighting' of the goal or target. In so open an environment the individual is vulnerable and needs to be guard against falling prey to the forces of greed, indifference, and cruelty.

9.3 SOLAR INFLUENCES

This the period of long nights and short days, the darkest month when the power of the Sun has departed and chilling winds herald the arrival of the first flurry of snow. But it is also a time of thanksgiving for the abundance that has been gathered and stored in preparation for the winter to come.

The waning solar energy, however, stimulates hope and encourages foresight and vision.

The related Sun sign is Sagittarius.

9.4 INFLUENCING WIND: West Winds
DIRECTION: North-west

The influence of the West Winds brings clarity of mind to those born in the Long Nights Time which is so necessary to cope with change and renewal. The West Winds have a keen edge which enables their direction to be more sharply defined and thereby help those who are born at this time to attain a clear sense of their own direction in life.

The West Winds are not strong and blustery and constantly changing their influence, but more penetrating and therefore stimulating and arousing the generation of inner Fire.

The north-west direction immediately precedes a cosmic 'gateway' at the entrance of the north-north-west, which on the Medicine Wheel was concerned with rebirth. In ancient northern European cultures it was celebrated as Yule around 22 December and 'recognized' the birth of cosmic consciousness. The north-west direction on the Wheel is a very potent place because it symbolizes 'initiation' as an essential preliminary to spiritual rebirth which some have described as 'Christ-consciousness'. Its polarity is in the south-east at the Flowering Time which precedes another cosmic 'gateway' which symbolized the entrance into human incarnation on the Medicine Wheel.

The north-west was the 'gateway' of initiation into the mysteries of life and in order to pass through it one had to demonstrate that one had learned correct use of the powers with which one had been entrusted. The greatest of these powers was the power of creative thought.

On the Medicine Wheel the north-west is also the place of karma where the unintegrated experiences of the past formulate patterns that are repeated into future lives until their lessons have been learned and applied.

The north-west direction is thus the direction for determining what to aim for and for learning how to take control of the constant movement of change.

Just as the *grizzly bear*, which is the totem animal of the West, is able to survive by its own strength, so the emphasis of the north-west is on self-reliance and on the power that comes from within. Its influence on those born in the Long Nights Time is in bringing out their potentials and hidden talents and enabling them to adapt to whatever environment or circum-stance in which they find themselves. Its emphasis is not so much on absorbing knowledge as on imparting it. It is a quality that enables many people born in the Long Nights Time to become excellent teachers.

9.5 INFLUENCING ELEMENTS: **Fire with Earth**

Elemental Earth helps stabilize and sustain, and this influence is vital in the realization of ideas and ideals. It is the influence of step-by-step progress that ensures there is a firm footing with each move forward. Its emphasis is on carefulness, but this has to be properly discerned. Otherwise it can develop into over-cautiousness and placidity.

Elemental Fire in its cyclical activity stimulates and inspires and provides the spark of idealism. It also motivates activity.

9.6 ELEMENTAL CLAN: **The Hawk (Fire) Clan**

People whose birthdays are from 23 November to 21 December are of the Hawk Clan and are generally bright and clear-sighted. They are motivated by an inner Fire that drives them on to new challenges and to become pioneers and leaders. Like Falcons and Salmon they need the warmth of firm friendships and close relationships.

9.7 Birth and Animal Totem: Owl

Owls are soft-feathered and short-tailed birds with large heads, flattened faces with enormous eyes, and partly hidden hooked beaks. They are nocturnal creatures and might be described as the night-time equivalent of hawks and falcons.

The barn owl is an effective and powerful totem. It has a white face, pale feathers and long legs. It lives alone or in pairs and roosts in hollow trees, church towers and farm buildings. It hunts at night and feeds mostly on small rodents.

The female barn owl lays four to seven eggs which take thirty-three days to incubate. During this time the male brings her food. Owls are caring about their young.

Although many people regard the owl as a creature of dark augury, this attitude stems from times when everything was done to denigrate what had previously been held sacred. In pre-Christian times the owl was associated with the mind and with wisdom and sacred science. It was a sacred bird.

Like their animal totem, Owl people conduct themselves proudly, and some even flamboyantly. Because they are so observant that little of relevance escapes their attention, they have a keen eye for detail and a good insight into whatever they set their minds on.

Owl people in general feel drawn to esoteric subjects and 'secret' things, but with this inquisitive urge is an intuitive 'pull' towards cautiousness and the need to keep themselves grounded in the world of practical reality.

This desire to vanish from view like the owl disappearing into the darkness is reflected in many way, sometimes by the normally outgoing Owl person becoming withdrawn, even to the point of avoiding the company of others, or sometimes breaking away from situations in which they have been supportive or deeply involved. It is during such times that the Owl person is in danger of being misunderstood and causing hurt to others as well as to themselves.

The owl is associated with wisdom that is 'hidden' and with light that shines in the darkness, like the Moon. The Owl person often finds themself being made aware of some way of the reality of a situation before its effects become obvious to others. This is a form of illumination which precedes any 'awakening' experience that is to follow.

9.8 PLANT TOTEM: Mistletoe

Mistletoe (*Phoradendron flavesceris* and *Viscum album*) is a semi-parasitic evergreen shrub that grows on various kinds of trees, notably apple, hawthorn and maple. It lives partly off its host tree and partly off food it obtains by its own chlorophyll. Both American and European mistletoe have thick, woody stems and leathery leaves. The flower-heads grow on spikes which fork into two. It bears white, fleshy berries which contain sticky seeds.

Indians regarded mistletoe as a kind of tree snake, and used it medicinally for cholera, convulsions and hysteria.

In Europe in olden times it was treated as a sacred plant for it heralded the beginning of the dark half of the year around the Autumn Equinox and reached its peak around the time of the Winter Solstice.

The way that mistletoe entwines itself around a tree was likened to the gentle embrace of a lover, and its translucent berries were likened to semen. Hence its association with love and fertility. Mistletoe was sometimes worn by women as an amulet to promote conception.

The Christmas-time practice of kissing under the mistletoe is an indication that it was considered to have certain 'magikal' properties which still live on in racial memory. Mistletoe is often associated with death and rebirth but its real significance concerns continuity of life.

Like their plant totem, Owl people have certain clinging qualities and even a 'magikal' air about them. The emphasis is on renewal.

9.9 MINERAL TOTEM: Obsidian

Obsidian is a glassy, solidified lava from a volcano that has fused so quickly that there are no crystals in it. The contains silica, aluminium and sometimes potassium, iron oxide and sodium. It is capable of being fashioned to provide a sharp cutting edge, and was often made into knives and arrowheads as well as jewellery.

Since obsidian comes from deep within the Earth, it is related to the inner nature of the human being, which can be very powerful and deserves to be respected.

The American Indian attributed obsidian with the power to sharpen both the outer and inner vision and with stimulating the foresight so that one could 'see' into the future.

Obsidian is translucent and usually black, and small spherical forms of obsidian are sometimes referred to as 'Apache Tears'. The name is derived from an incident in Arizona when a band of Pineal Apaches were ambushed by military regulars. Most were killed and the survivors, rather than submit, threw themselves over a cliff edge. Tears were shed by the women and maidens of the tribe at the base of the cliff for a moon, and a legendary tale says that the tears were embedded into black stones and that whoever possessed one of these 'Apache tears' would never themselves suffer grave sorrow.

Apache Tears are said to balance the emotions and to be a protection against emotional traumas. Certainly they are a powerful meditation tool.

Owl people can be like obsidian – shiny and bright but with a sharp edge to their nature which enables them to cut right through to the heart of things. Owl people should wear obsidian, for it is considered a protection against harmful influences.

9.10 POLARITY TOTEM: Deer

Owls are determined and fearless and difficult to budge once they have made up their minds. Their protectiveness has a tendency to block off their innermost feelings so they may shy away from relationships which might make them feel vulnerable.

Owls can gain assurance from Deer people who have a similar proud and discerning attitude but with it a sensitivity to the needs of others which is borne out by their intuitiveness and resourcefulness, qualities which Owls need to develop.

9.11 PERSONALITY EXPRESSION
Adult

Warm-hearted, jovial, fun-loving, Owl has a lively mind, an independent outlook and an adventurous temperament. They like the great outdoors and its freedom from confinement and limitation. Owls require freedom of mind and expression, and freedom to go where they please, think what they like and say what they feel. Their minds are so alert that they are inclined to develop more interests than they can cope with and thus become masters of none.

Their enquiring minds entice them into lengthy discussions and arguments. They enjoy talking about things that interest them at the time, but are less enthusiastic about other people's interests.

Owls are individualistic and sincere and have a jovial disposition, but they are prone to making explosive expressions if they are touched on a raw spot, and to bouts of anger if they are provoked. Their boldness and frankness can sometimes come across as insensitivity or just plain rudeness, and they can be bitterly sarcastic when hurt.

Although Owls require freedom of movement, they can sometimes run away from their responsibilities in a blind dash to avoid burdensome problems. Usually, such attempts to evade responsibility rebound on them, and problems and ties increase rather than diminish.

Physically Owls are courageous and are usually attracted to dangerous sports because risk and recklessness exhilarates them.

Owls are adventurous and enjoy opening up new ways that others may follow. They are pioneers, explorers and visionaries, and they like doing things in a big way, though they are rarely satisfied. They will always come back for more, and when that appetite is for material things they can find it difficult to discern between need and greed.

For all their exuberance and confidence, Owls find themselves pursuing many blind alleys and dissipating their energies in all too many directions so that their plans and ambitions rarely materialize completely. They need to learn to fix their mind on a single, clear goal for they have the energy and determination to attain it.

Positive traits: Jovial. Versatile. Philosophical. Adaptable. Scrupulous. Dependable.

Negative traits: Extremism. Tactlessness. Restlessness. Boisterousness. Capriciousness.

Vocational possibilities: Arts. Law. Writing. Librarianship. Music. Public speaking. Selling. Politics. Theology.

Child

The Owl infant craves company. It will cry when left on its own, but gurgle contentedly within a few minutes of being brought into a room where there are others. It just likes the reassurance of the herd.

Owl children have a happy-go-lucky nature and enjoy the fun of joining in things. They have a quite taxing sense of curiosity and their questions invariably begin with 'Why?'.

Parent

Owls are usually bored with the routine and graft of child-rearing and can be pretty lax on discipline, but their children usually respond well to their active and adventurous interest as they get older.

The Owl father is a great encouragement to his offspring interested in sports and outdoor pursuits and will get fully involved with the children.

The Owl mother is devoted to her children but is rarely possessive. Indeed, as the children get older she acts more like a big sister and a genuine friend.

9.12 ROMANCE AND SEX

Owls are flirtatious romantics. They enjoy all the thrills and spills of falling in love, but they don't like the idea of being fettered. Being tied down terrifies them, and they usually take their time before making any long-term commitment. When they do, love-making has to be adventurous and exciting and then they will be ardent lovers. If it loses its thrill and excitement, sex turns into a bore and then a chore.

Compatibilities: Owls are compatible with Falcons (21 March – 19 April) and Salmon (22 July – 21 August).

Spiritual sexuality: The spiritual sexuality is essentially masculine – thrusting and energetic.

9.13 HEALTH

Owl's appetite for the good things of life – especially food and drink – can put a strain on the waistline and the liver. Since the hips and thighs are the most vulnerable area of Owls, it is these that are likely to suffer the burden of excessive weight.

There is always the problems of nervous exhaustion through taking on too much.

9.14 AFFINITY COLOUR: Gold

Gold is a colour and a metal and though it draws impurities to itself it is refined by fire (the fire of adversity?) and so becomes more valuable.

Gold, as a higher octave of orange, radiates love and compassion. It is the colour of realization and the striving for perfection. Positively applied its emphasis is inspiring and comforting. Negatively applied it can lead to self-indulgence and greed.

Gold represents that which is enduring and the very essence of life which does not tarnish. It is a colour that radiates warmth, vitality and well-being.

Gold stresses Owl's determined search for realization and perfection.

9.15 ADVANTAGEOUS TIMES

Best months of the year for Owl are from 21 March to 19 April, 22 July to 21 August, and 23 November to 21 December.

Best day of the week is Thursday.

Best times of the day are from 7 a.m. to 9 a.m. and 7 p.m. to 9 p.m.

9.16 OUTWARD (CONSCIOUS) AIM AND
INNER (SUBCONSCIOUS) DESIRE

The outward aim of the Owl is understanding. Owls are motivated by a need to search for meaning, particularly that which lies behind the externals and behind the experience. To the Owl there must be a meaning in everything.

On the inner level Owls are seeking to determine intent. This requires looking ahead in deciding what to aim for. So owls will be endeavouring to extend their vision and to broaden their horizons and by this means expand their spiritual development.

9.17 SPIRITUAL ALCHEMY

Owl is influenced by the elements of Earth and Fire, but it is Earth Fire – the planetary Fire – that provides the fervour and enthusiasm and that emotional warmth of Owl. Planetary Fire produces fervour and warmth in the emotional body, liveliness and wit in the mental body, and enterprise and initiative in the personality.

As Owls are born in a time that precedes a pivotal point in the Wheel, there is also a magnetic pull towards the direction of change which is from west to north, from Earth to Air. It is the pull of Air that gives them their desire for freedom of movement.

The directional influence is from cool to cold (– –) and the elemental pull is Earth (–) and Fire (+) and with an attraction towards Air (+). The spiritual sexuality is masculine (+). There is thus a balance between the active and thrusting and the attraction to the inner life. The combination is thus (– –, – + and +, and balanced with + by the attraction towards Air).

9.18 LIFE-CHALLENGES

Owls want freedom of movement and the liberty of conscience, but freedom in evading responsibilities which is sometimes sought is an escape that rebounds, for the laws of karma ensure that the responsibilities will arise again, reappearing perhaps in other forms and in different circumstance, but with the same old lessons to be learned. To be free does not mean running away from responsibilities and to be without problems. It

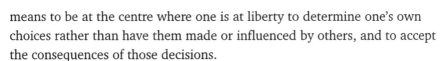

means to be at the centre where one is at liberty to determine one's own choices rather than have them made or influenced by others, and to accept the consequences of those decisions.

Owls are likely to find themselves frequently in situations where they are forced to consider the direction their lives are taking and to determine themselves what they want to do and where they want to go, rather than to become the victims of fate.

Part of the purpose of life for Owls is the recognition that direction emanates from thought and that thought supplies the power of direction, so the greatest power any human being can possess is the power of creative thought.

For all their exuberance and confidence, Owls find themselves pursuing many blind alleys and dissipating their energies so that their plans and ambitions rarely materialize completely. They must learn to fix their minds on one clear target at a time. The most powerful Red Indian warrior was not the one who could fire off the most arrows, but the one who concentrated his mind on a single target and whose aim was true.

Must cultivate: Optimism. Inspiration. Concentration.

Must avoid: Greed. Gluttony. Exaggeration. Over-indulgence.

9.19 PRIMARY FUNCTION AND LIFE-PATH

The Path of Owl is intended to lead to the discovery that whatever is required outwardly must first exist inwardly. That which is Without was first that which was Within.

The prime purpose is for the tempering of opposites in order to attain good management of one's potentials.

In the American Indian culture the weaving of a blanket required the mingling of many skills. It was treasured as a gift because it represented in an enduring form the inner beauty of the one who had woven it. It symbolized, too, the necessity for a balanced heart and mind and the need for rational thought to be balanced with feeling that comes from the heart. That is the path of Owl.

The primary function of Owl is elevation and exaltation. It requires opportunities for raising the intellect and elevating the morality to obtain the clarity of vision that is spirit insight.

9.20 THE I CHING TRIGRAM: Ken. The Still Mountain.

Owl is in the north-west position on the Wheel of the Year.

The Still Mountain symbolizes elevation, steadfastness and inner peace. It stresses the need to be still and to calm the mind in order to focus attention on the target. It emphasizes the importance of withdrawal, meditation and concentration.

9.21 HOW TO COPE WITH OWLS

Be sure of your facts. Discuss things fully with Owls. They aren't easily swayed, so any proposition has to be factually watertight.

Never indicate that you doubt Owl's good intentions.

Goose

SUMMARY

Birth dates:	22 December – 19 January (21 June – 21 July in the Southern hemisphere).
Earth influence:	The Renewal Time.
Influencing wind:	The North Winds. *Totem*: Buffalo.
Direction:	North-north-west.
Predominant elements:	Earth with Air.
Elemental clan:	Turtle (Earth) Clan. *Function*: preparing the ground.
Birth and animal totem:	Goose.
Plant totem:	Bramble.
Mineral totem:	Peridot.
Polarity totem:	Woodpecker.
Affinity colour:	White.
Personality:	Self-demanding. Reliable. Prudent. Austere.
Feelings:	Self-centred.
Intention:	Trust.
Nature:	Severe.
Positive traits:	Ambitious. Determined. Persevering.
Negative traits:	Rigid. Pessimistic. Demanding. Selfish.
Sex-drive:	Sensual and long-lasting.
Compatibilities:	Beavers, Brown Bears and Crows.
Conscious aim:	Conservation.
Subconscious desire:	Integrity.
Life-path:	Adaptation.
I Ching trigram:	☶ Ken. The Still Mountain. Courage and determination.
Must cultivate:	Sociability. Effective self-expression.
Must avoid:	Self-doubt. Pessimism.
Spiritual alchemy:	Yin predominates.
Starting totems:	Goose. Buffalo. Turtle. Bramble. Peridot. Woodpecker.

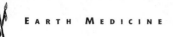

10. Goose

10.1 BIRTH MONTH: 22 December – 19 January

10.2 EARTH INFLUENCE: The Renewal Time

This is the first cycle of winter and contains the Winter Solstice which brings with it a time for refreshment and renewal.

People born at this time are practical and ambitious and though they like to have people around them are reluctant to let relationships develop beyond the superficial. Though they have a liking for people, they may appear to be reserved, and this is because they feel emotionally vulnerable if they give too much of themselves to others.

10.3 SOLAR INFLUENCES

At the beginning of the month, the shortest day and longest night of the Winter Solstice marks a potent stage in the yearly cycle. The Sun appears to have departed for good and the Earth lies barren and dormant, cold and neglected, and everywhere in Nature is the air of austerity.

Yet the darkest day is the herald of glad tidings, for that which appeared to have departed is reborn and will begin to wax again and the turn of the Wheel of Life will soon indicate the new life which is now promised.

The seeds of the new life are stirring within the womb of the Earth, though their quickening is not yet apparent.

In northern Europe in ancient times, Yule was the joyous celebration of that which is dead but is now alive, or rebirth and renewal, of the beginning of a new cycle in the pattern of life. It was the Festival of Rebirthing which symbolized the coming back to life not just of the physical Sun, which was only a symbol, but the newly risen sun of one's own individual self.

This festival was replaced by the Christian Christmas to commemorate the birth of Christ which some scholars think took place at a different time of the year (September), but the spirit of goodwill, of family gatherings, feasting and merrymaking, continues to this day.

The related Sun sign is Capricorn.

10.4 INFLUENCING WIND: The North Winds

The North Winds are associated with purity and renewal and are at their most powerful when the Earth lies dormant and in the grip of winter. It is a time when man and animal seek shelter and warmth from the wind's sharp and penetrating 'bite' and withdraw from external activities to turn inward and to look forward to the warmer and brighter days to come.

The influence of the North Winds is paradoxical for it is not seen solely as the cold air that turns water into ice or causes the ice crystals to dance on the leaves of the evergreen trees. It is a hidden, internalized power that works unseen and unfelt. It is the power whose energy penetrates down into the dormant seed that lies 'asleep' beneath the Earth's hard and frozen surface but is being purified and prepared so that it will be seen to burst into new life when the Sun returns to cover the Earth in a warm embrace.

The North Winds, then, encourage patience and inward growth, and renewal of the mind and body. They help, too, to establish purity of intent and purpose.

This power of the North was represented by some Indian tribes by the totem of the *buffalo*. In times when the survival of a tribe was dependent on hunting, the buffalo roamed much of North America in great herds. Not only did it supply meat for food, but its hide provided material for the tipis in which people lived, and the clothes they wore, and its bones were made into the implements they used. The buffalo thus gave totally of itself so that the people could be renewed completely and for this reason it was revered above all animals.

The power of the North was seen as the great renewing force of sustenance and security and which was effective on all levels of existence. It is the power of a renewed mind, refreshed and alert and fast-acting after sleep and empowered with knowledge and wisdom. It is the power of a body beautiful, nourished and strengthened after sustenance. It is the power of a revived spirit, free to wander and explore and experience without limitation.

The power of the North is seen as the power that brings new thoughts, new ideas, and newness of life.

10.5 INFLUENCING ELEMENTS: Earth with Air

Air is the element that is associated with the mind, with thoughts and ideas, and with raid and sometimes unexpected change and movement. Whereas Fire energizes, Water refreshes, and Earth sustains, Air enlivens and transforms. It is elemental Air that is seen as the influence that enables things to be transformed and accomplished through the power of new ideas and dreams.

Like elemental Air, people born in the Renewal Time are quick, sharp and adaptable, with an ability to perform the unexpected. They are always active and on the move.

Elemental Earth brings the pull towards stability and security and with it the characteristics of predictability and dependability.

10.6 ELEMENTAL CLAN: Turtle (Earth) Clan

People whose birthdays are between 22 December and 19 January are born into the Turtle Clan and affected by the stability of the Earth element. Solidity, security, dependability, predictability – all these are qualities of importance to Turtle Clan people. To them word and deed are aspects of the same thing, so generally they are true to their word and become upset when others fail to do what they have said they would do.

Turtle Clan people can be self-sacrificing and once they have made up their minds about what they want, they will stick rigidly to a course of action.

10.7 BIRTH AND ANIMAL TOTEM: Goose

Geese are large birds with long necks and short legs and fly in large flocks making a loud honking noise. Their habitat is on moors and marshes and grassland near lakes and rivers and though they are good swimmers they feed mainly off the land.

The goose was a favourite totem among the Celts of pre-Christian Britain, and its appearance as a major character in European fairy-stories (Mother Goose; the Goose that laid the Golden Egg, etc.) is indicative of its significant place in ancient lore, for fairy-stories and folk-tales contain the essence of the symbology of the esoteric teachings of long ago.

The high-flying goose honking its way across the midwinter skies was associated with the powers of the North, which are described elsewhere, and with the act of purification and renewal. Indeed, the traditional Christmas meal of goose may well have had its roots in a ritual feast of sacred goose flesh which emphasized the process of renewal.

There are many species of geese, but one revered by American Indians was the snowgoose, so named not just because of its snow-white plumage, but because its life on the North American continent appeared to be governed by the snow.

Indians referred to the snowgoose as 'the bird from beyond the north winds' because it migrated from its nesting grounds in the far north of the Arctic when snow began to fall in the autumn and did not return until the snow vanished in early spring.

Like all geese, the snowgoose flies in flocks but during its migration these flocks are vast, sometimes numbering several thousand.

Some are said to travel 5,000 miles each year to and from their nesting grounds in the northern Arctic.

Like their totem, people born during the Renewal Time have imaginative minds that enable them to traverse new frontiers and to set out on long-term aims.

Goose people are perfectionists and, like their totem, are prone to nit-picking, letting comparatively minor issues bother them. When they allow themselves to feel low because of an obstacle in their path or because their dreams seem a long way from fulfilment, they can become really melancholy and bring a blanket of gloom and despondency all around them.

When in a positive frame of mind, they can surprise others by the sheer energy of their endeavours and with their bubbling enthusiasm.

The goose is white, the colour of purity, a quality which is emphasized prominently in the lives of Goose people for when it is expressed as purity of *intent*, the seemingly impossible becomes attainable for them.

In Amerindian symbology the goose was regarded as a Great Dreamer. This quality is reflected also in Goose people, whose aspirations inspire them to do ordinary things extra-ordinarily well, even to perfection.

Goose people have intrinsic gifts which enable them to be good teachers of children, especially of the handicapped, and they will find fulfilment in any work which involves them with children or with the handicapped or mentally retarded.

Silver Bear explained to me that Goose people carry around with them a reflection of their Higher Self. He meant that they have clear aspirations and a determination to fulfil what they see in their mind's eye. They find frustration mainly because their dreams cannot be fulfilled speedily.

10.8 PLANT TOTEM: Bramble

The bramble (*Rubus villosus*), commonly called the blackberry or dewberry, is a perennial trailing plant which has slender branches with sharp prickles. The serrated leaves have fine hairs. The plant carries white five-petalled flowers from July to September and bears its fruits in the autumn.

Indians used the roots and leaves medicinally as a remedy for diarrhoea, and a tea made from the dried leaves was used to treat enteritis and colic. Bramble leaves were also chewed to heal bleeding gums.

The prickly thorns of the bramble denote both protection and suffering, both qualities which Goose people seem to experience in some abundance during their lives, often encountering difficulties and danger which cause them pain, yet seeming to be protected from any permanent harm.

As a midwinter totem for the time of the Winter Solstice and the 'death' of the Sun, the transformational aspect of the bramble is perhaps being emphasized, suggesting that entanglement and suffering must sometimes be experienced in order for us to bear our ripest fruit. As fertile fruits of Mother Earth, bramble berries were said to confer inspiration, a special quality of the North, so this totem is concerned very much with inspiration and the courage and persistence that is often required in order to reach it.

10.9 MINERAL TOTEM: **Peridot**

Peridot is a magnesium-iron silicate found in igneous rocks and is also called chrysolite or olivine. It is a delicate green stone with a glassy lustre and the clear varieties are cut as gemstones.

The Amerindians regarded it as petrified 'heavenly' radiance that came direct from the Sun force and as a stone of light was related to clear-sightedness and to clarity of mind. It was also related to the spiritual Sun so it was considered to be a stone to impart spiritual strength and spiritual discernment. Peridot is thus linked with intuitive insight and inner vision, and with the ability to see into the future.

Peridot has a soothing sensitivity especially if worn in a headdress or at the base of the throat for it is reputed to affect the chakras in the head.

10.10 POLARITY TOTEM: **Woodpecker**

Goose people have an eye for detail and an inner striving for perfection, but they are often thrown off balance by little things and by the slightest provocation. They have an inherent resistance to sudden change, preferring to make haste slowly, so they sometimes find it difficult to cope with the unexpected and with the failings they see in others which they allow to affect their own lives.

They can draw lessons in coping with such difficulties by looking to Woodpecker who emphasizes the importance of having a secure and harmonious base and the need to share with others. This, of course, can be interpreted in a spiritual sense for the quest to find spiritual direction and perfection has to be balanced with a sense of security, and love, to be received, must first be given.

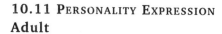

10.11 PERSONALITY EXPRESSION
Adult

Determined, ambitious, practical, resourceful Goose. People born in the Renewal Time have plenty of vigour in pursuing their own interests, but generally prefer to keep themselves from becoming too involved in the lives of others.

This aloofness does not mean that Goose people are uncaring. They are truly concerned for their loved ones and for those whose loyalty and dependability have survived the test of time, but they do have a wariness of getting too involved with others, and though they may have associations with many there will be few they could call friends.

Goose people are able to draw from an inner reservoir of strength which enables them to work untiringly, and to be unflinching about depriving themselves of many of life's pleasures. And even to suffer hardship for a time in order to attain a heart's desire. This ability to tap a source of inner strength enables them to develop a shrewdness to recognize the true value of things and to turn adverse circumstances into their ultimate advantage.

Although born at a time of the year which is the most barren, Goose people have a love of Nature and of all creatures that sometimes appears to exceed their concern for the welfare of humans.

They have an idealism which causes them to take things too seriously, and perhaps to get some problems out of proportion, with the result that they become highly strung and tense. They are prone to bouts of pessimism and gloominess when things get on top of them and they feel mistreated and misunderstood. If they allow this trend to develop they can become sour and embittered and then any provocation can cause them to be quite destructive.

The goose is certainly a tough old bird, but it has a tender and gentle heart.

Positive traits: Ambitious. Determined. Reliable. Prudent. Patient. Persevering.

Negative traits: Pessimistic. Mean. Conventional. Demanding. Selfish.

Vocational possibilities: Agriculture. Arts. Banking. Economics. Commerce. Collecting. Farming. Dancing. Law. Politics. Military. Trading. Mortician.

Child

Goose babies are sweet and good-tempered with a strange knowingness about them which makes the baby-talk of grown-ups seem out of place.

As infants, and during their early years at school, they may appear timid and bashful, lacking in the confidence of most of their peers. They may appear reluctant even to join in games and might even be described as poor mixers. However, as they grow older it becomes clear that they can be trusted with responsibility and often turn out to be running things for others.

They are usually neat and tidy children and, indeed, can become quite distressed by disorder of any kind.

Parent

Goose people are not usually enthusiastic parents. It is not that they are uncaring or irresponsible. It is just that they are happier when children do things for themselves rather than being entirely dependent.

Their offspring certainly don't get pampered. Goose parents like to have their children follow a routine and expect them to behave properly and to show good manners.

10.12 ROMANCE AND SEX

Goose people want the security and protection of a lasting partnership. They are, therefore, less prone to love at first sight. For them, love is more likely to develop from a long-lasting friendship than from a casual meeting.

They are unlikely to show their affection openly, but in private they can be sensual and passionate lovers. They need to feel safe and secure before they respond. As in everything Goose does, it has to do well and sex is no exception. Geese are capable and understanding lovers and have a great deal of stamina and staying power.

Goose men are good providers, dependable and faithful. Goose women are fine home-makers and quite brilliant with the housekeeping.

Compatibilities: Goose people are compatible with Beavers (those born between 20 April and 20 May), Brown Bears (22 August to 21 September) and Crow (22 September to 22 October).

10.13 HEALTH

Goose people have a strong constitution. They don't give in easily to illness of any kind, but will soldier on long after most people suffering similarly would have taken to their beds.

Nervous rashes and allergies are common among Goose people and these are often brought on through suppression of their emotions. They also have a tendency to suffer from knee problems and knee injuries and rheumatic complaints.

10.14 AFFINITY COLOUR: White

White is a reflector of other colours, and is a symbol of purity and psychic energy. It indicates simplicity and purity of intent.

Goose people send out thoughts and impressions which affect other people. A good proportion of Goose people are regarded as psychic. They are prone to an excessiveness which makes them rather difficult to live with.

10.15 ADVANTAGEOUS TIMES

Best months of the year for Goose people are from 22 December to 19 January, 20 April to 20 May, and 22 August to 21 September.
Best day of the week is Saturday.
Best times of the day are from 9 a.m. to 11 a.m. and 9 p.m. to 11 p.m.

10.16 OUTWARD (CONSCIOUS) AIM AND INNER (SUBCONSCIOUS) DESIRE

The outward (conscious) aim of Goose is to organize and conserve, but the inner drive is towards purification. This is much more than purification in a moralistic sense. The emphasis is on the need to become self-reliant and self-sufficient and the establishment of individual self-identity.

It is likely that those born in the Renewal Time will undergo many traumatic and testing experiences and suffer some spiritual loneliness, all of which will put a heavy demand on them. Such experiences are part of a transforming process that is bringing the individual to a state of becoming more 'complete'. It is a renewal process that is concerned with developing the spiritual muscles to climb to the mountain top.

10.17 SPIRITUAL ALCHEMY

Goose people are materialistic through the influence of elemental Earth, but they are the most changeable of those influenced also by elemental Air. They have a tenacity and quality of endurance associated with Earth but the influence of Air drives them on with boundless energy in spite of what sometimes seem to be insurmountable obstacles.

The directional polarity is cold (– –), the elemental polarities are Air + and Earth –. The spiritual sexuality is feminine (–). The combination is thus decidedly receptive and introverted with the personality being constantly thrown back into itself. The combination is (– –, + – and –).

10.18 Life-Challenges

The life of Goose is one of persistence and hard work in a constant endeavour to find security. Every success will be hard-earned.

During the most crucial times Goose may appear to be hemmed in by restrictions and limitations and by the obstructive tactics of others, but each should be seen as a challenge which if approached constructively will lead to expansion and true achievement. No obstacle encountered by Geese is greater than their own self-doubt and pessimism.

10.19 Primary Function and Life-Path

The primary function of Goose is to bring to completion – to develop things fully.

The life-path is one of adaptation. There is a trite old saying, 'Bend lest you break' which is particularly appropriate to Goose. The path is one of perfection in the sense of completion. When this principle is applied moralistically – particularly in judging the attitudes and actions of others – it becomes an obstruction on the path and creates a barrier to progress.

Goose has an innate urge for freedom, but to attain that state confining attitudes must be willingly abandoned in order to be released from the attachments of the past. Goose often presents a face to the world that is far removed from how they really are. Coming into freedom is where there is no longer a need for pretence.

The prime purpose of being on this path is to attain understanding. But understanding is that which cannot be learned or developed or even attained through the passage of time. It comes in an instant. It is a matter of being prepared to receive it.

10.20 The I Ching Trigram: Ken. The Still Mountain.

People born during Renewal Time are on the north-north-west position on the Wheel of the Year.

In this trigram, the rugged rocky terrain of a mountain is presented as a challenge – the challenge of awesome territory that must be conquered and claimed. It exemplifies courage and determination.

10.21 How to Cope with Geese

Goose people are essentially practical and materialistic, so be down-to-earth. Don't interrupt them when they are hard at work.

Goose people rarely respond to emotional appeal and dislike anything that smells of insincerity.

Otter

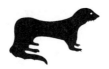

Summary

Birth dates:	20 January – 18 February (22 July – 21 August in the Southern hemisphere).
Earth influence:	The Cleansing Time.
Influencing wind:	The North Winds. *Totem:* Buffalo.
Direction:	North.
Predominant element:	Air.
Elemental clan:	Butterfly (Air) Clan. *Function:* to carry through.
Birth and animal totem:	Otter.
Plant totem:	Fern.
Mineral totem:	Turquoise.
Polarity totem:	Salmon.
Affinity colour:	Silver.
Personality:	Jovial. Friendly. Unconventional. Independent. Dynamic.
Feelings:	Detached.
Intention:	Imagination.
Nature:	Humanitarian.
Positive traits:	Inventive. Reforming. Perceptive.
Negative traits:	Unpredictable. Rebellious. Tactless. Eccentric.
Sex-drive:	Hot and cold.
Compatibilities:	Crows, Falcons and Deer.
Conscious aim:	Knowledge.
Subconscious desire:	Wisdom.
Life-path:	Creative strength.
I Ching trigram:	☴ Sun. The Gentle Wind. Flexible vision.
Must cultivate:	Inventiveness. Tolerance. Courage.
Must avoid:	Rebelliousness. Eccentricity.
Spiritual alchemy:	Yin predominates.
Starting totems:	Otter. Buffalo. Butterfly. Fern. Turquoise. Salmon.

11. Otter

11.1 BIRTH MONTH: 20 January – 18 February

11.2 EARTH INFLUENCE: The Cleansing Time

This middle cycle of the winter season is the time when the Earth is cleansing itself before the pace of life increases and things begin to grow again.

Its key emphasis is preparation, so people born at this time are planners and innovators and visionaries with perceptive and intuitive natures.

People born in the Cleansing Time are learning the lessons of formulating things and of discovering ways of service. They are the preservers and conservationists.

11.3 SOLAR INFLUENCES

This midpoint in the winter season is when the solar influence is stirring and its electrical energy is beginning to be evident in the freshness of the air itself which is stimulating, invigorating and cleansing. It is the power that is breaking through the grip of limitations and constraints.

There are stirrings, too, within the Womb of Mother Earth, as the new life that is to come is moving into manifestation but hidden beneath the surface.

In many ancient cultures these first stirrings of Nature were celebrated by a festival in early February. In Britain it was known as Imbolc, a Gaelic name which means 'in the belly' implying 'quickening'. It celebrated the return of light. It was replaced later by its Christian equivalent of Candlemass on 2 February.

Anciently, it was a festival of cleansing, of clearing the ground of dead growth, of clearing out the clutter of things that accumulated during the winter and were no longer needed. It was the origin of spring-cleaning. It was the preparation time for new growth which would be springing into being soon when the dormancy of winter burst into the sudden activity of spring.

The Amerindians related such cleansing and clearing with the ceremony of the Give-Away – an occasion for giving away those things in life that one wanted to get rid of – the banishment of bad attitudes and habits, petty fears and jealousies, and ill feelings. Symbolically each was represented by a single grain or by a stick that was cast into the fire and consumed.

The related Sun sign is Aquarius.

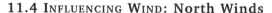

11.4 Influencing Wind: North Winds
Direction: North

In the Northern hemisphere, the Sun does not appear in the north, going from east through south-west, and the sky appears to revolve around the North Star, so the North was regarded as the mysterious hub around which the heavens turned, and as the power of the unseen.

The power of the North was the power of new life that is hidden in rest, the power that turns water to ice, and the power ofd ice that breaks mighty rocks into small pebbles.

The power of the North indicated the need to be silent and to listen, to get away from chatter and confusion, and hustle and bustle. So it is associated with meditation and contemplation whose essence is to rest from external activity so that one can provide opportunity for inner growth.

The Amerindians associated the North with knowledge and wisdom and with the power of thought, and the north winds with mental activity. The totem is the *buffalo* (see 10.4).

11.5 Influencing Element: Air

Air is the element associated with the intellect and with the power of thought, for the idea or the thoughts precedes manifestation or creation.

Air is clear and uncluttered and is so likened to the visualization of creative thought, and Air is unseen movement so it can be likened also to the impetus of the unmanifest becoming manifest, of that which is invisible coming into visibility.

It is through the movement of Air that we are aware of sound, of hearing and being heard. So it is through Air that it is possible to communicate with others. Air is thus linked with communication.

Communication, ideas, mental activity, creativity – all these things will be much in evidence among those born in the Cleansing Time for elemental Air has a powerful influence in all areas of their lives.

11.6 Elemental Clan: Butterfly (Air) Clan

People born between 20 January and 18 February are born into the Butterfly Clan, which is the clan of elemental Air which enables them to transform and rejuvenate conditions and other people by the freshness of their approach and by their activities.

They can, however, dissipate their energies by flitting from one thing to another, and by sudden and unexpected changes of direction, and their state of constant motion can cause them to overtax themselves.

Once they have established a sense of direction their lives can be both stimulating and fulfilling.

11.7 Birth and Animal Totem: Otter

The principal totem for those born in the Cleansing Time is the *otter*. The otter is a member of the weasel family and is at home on both land and water. It has a thick, powerful tail that is tapered to serve as a rudder in water and as a tool for use in the otter's construction work. The otter has short, strong legs and webbed feet which enable it to swim speedily through water. It is able to stay underwater for up to four minutes.

The otter has a long body which, fully grown, can be up to 90 cm (3 ft) long. It lives mainly on fish. The otter is noted for its sense of fun and its play. Its home is a hole in the riverbank with an underwater entrance.

Because the otter can adopt postures which are considered unusual in animals, it is regarded as something of a mimic.

The otter has a strong sense of family and is ardent towards its companions, often mourning the death of a mate for a long time afterwards. The young cubs stay longer with their parents than the offspring of most animals.

Like the animal totem, people born at this time of the year are usually friendly, helpful, playful and bold. Their spirit of helpfulness is such that they often engage themselves in charitable activities. They, too, can be good at mimicking others.

The emphasis in the lives of Otter people is service. They are considerate and many of their life-experiences will present ways in which their energies can be directed to the benefit of the Earth and its inhabitants. Should this be blocked for whatever reason, or should they allow themselves to become too self-centred, they are likely to become miserable and morose.

Just as the otter is one of the great organisers of the animal kingdom, so Otter people excel at running things in the human kingdom. And just as the otter keeps the water in which it lives very clean, so Otter people require cleanliness and orderliness in both their home and working environment; otherwise they feel uncomfortable and ill at ease.

11.8 Plant Totem: Fern

Polipody is a common name for female fern (*Polypodium vulgare*) which is a perennial evergreen plant that grows profusely in shady areas, in

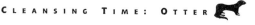

woodlands and among rocks. Its leaves, or fronds, vary considerably in length and taper to a point. They grow from the top of a root-like stem which creeps along or just below the surface.

Spore cases grow in two rows on either side of the mid-vein on the underside of the leaves. These mature from a yellowish to a bright orange colour in late autumn.

Indians used the rootstock to make an infusion to treat coughs and respiratory problems, and also as a cleanser to wash external wounds.

The male fern (*Dryopteris filix-mus*) is a coarser and more upright plant. Among its medicinal uses was as a remedy for tapeworms.

Like their plant totem, Otter people have a capacity to bend with the wind and to be adaptable though persistent. They are likely to suffer stress if their tendency is blocked in any way.

11.9 MINERAL TOTEM: Turquoise

Turquoise is a soft, sky-blue or green-blue stone with a wax-like lustre. It contains copper and aluminium phosphates with silica, ammonia and water.

It is a sensitive stone which is said to absorb harmful vibrations and loses its colour if its wearer is unwell or in any kind of physical danger. It will sometimes shatter under vibrational strain, and because of this characteristic some Amerindians wore turquoise to protect them from injury and especially from breaking bones for they believed that the turquoise itself would fracture instead. Some Indians decorated their horses' tails or bridles with turquoise as a protection against the animal breaking a limb in a fall.

The blue turquoise was often referred to as the 'stone of the sky', meaning the mystical realm. Otter people may find themselves attracted to mystical things, and their life-experiences will be drawing them to learn to balance the physical with the spiritual.

The turquoise was considered to enhance the understanding. It has an energy pattern of great vitality which affects the mental body and brings a sense of calm and peacefulness because it is such a good balancer of energies. An Otter person should wear turquoise since they are especially vulnerable to the wiles of others and to emotional disturbance. Turquoise will help them to retain their balance under pressure.

Turquoise stones worn as a bracelet on the left wrist can enhance the owner's healing abilities. Used in meditation, turquoise can bring out the purpose and meaning of any situation.

11.10 Polarity Totem: Salmon

Otter people generally have a genuine concern for the well-being of fellow humans and involve themselves in charitable and humanitarian projects. This desire to serve is an inherent part of their nature. They are also dreamers and visionaries, and these qualities need to be balanced with practicality.

Otters can learn from Salmon, who are similarly sympathetic to the needs of others, but also have a capacity to develop a thick skin to protect parts of their sensitive nature from those who might try to manipulate or control them.

11.11 Personality Expression
Adult

Artistic, independent, humane, dynamic, constructive Otter. Otter people are outgoing and like to be involved with people for they regard everyone as a friend. They have a deep love of freedom and independence, and they support equality of the sexes, equal opportunity for all, and fair treatment for people of all races and creeds. They resent any form of enforced obedience and find it hard to conform to rules and regulations.

They have flair and originality, but often their schemes and ideas are impractical or utopian. Otter people have busy minds and are often pre-occupied with plans that they do not have the time to fulfil. They are prone to taking on commitments which they are far too busy to meet.

Otter people are broad-minded and have few taboos and prejudices and will try almost anything. Experimentation is a way of finding out for themselves, and for this reason they may appear rather eccentric. They are inventive and have a flair for originality, and are unpredictable.

Idealistic, they have a reforming zeal which may be regarded as revolutionary but never in a destructive way.

Otter people approach all their problems analytically, and almost clinically, for while they have empathy for others and are affected by their emotions, these rarely run very deep. Though they like being involved with others they like to be personally detached.

They have a lively temperament which most people find likeable, and an intuitive insight which enables them to be particularly perceptive. They are self-assured and usually self-reliant.

Positive traits: Friendly. Willing. Inventive. Reforming. Lively. Perceptive.

Negative traits: Unpredictable. Eccentric. Tactless. Rebellious. Self-centred.

Vocational possibilities: Arts. Archaeology. Astronomy. Electronics.

Invention. Medicine. Psychology. Psychiatry. Philosophy. Teaching.
Scientific research. Writing.

Child

The Otter is a loveable and often amusing baby, but is unpredictable. Otter
infants can turn off their apparent docility and become so demanding
they'll have Mum and Dad chasing around in all directions.

They don't stay babies for long, and are usually ahead of other infants
in their development. At school they demonstrate their agile minds in most
subjects, but sometimes find difficulty in organizing their thoughts and
remembering what they have learned. They need encouragement to take
part in physical activities and when they do they can be quite good at
almost any sport.

Parent

Otter parents usually develop a friendly and open relationship with their
children and encourage them to talk about their problems and difficulties.
It is part of the process of helping the child become independent.

The Otter father gets involved in his children's activities, and gets so
engrossed in the fun that he behaves like a kid himself. But he's equally
involved in helping junior with the homework.

The Otter woman is usually a devoted mother, though her tolerant
attitude and reticence in demonstrating her affections makes her seem
rather detached. She is, however, helpful and reassuring to her offspring
and tender and gentle when they're ill.

11.12 ROMANCE AND SEX

Otters blow hot and cold when it comes to love. They're interested in the
mind more than the body, but none the less can be electrifying lovers.
Their problem is that their idealism causes them not only to want the
perfect mate, but to imagine themselves as the perfect lover. So while they
may have lots of ideas about sex, their own lack of intense emotion and
passion may result in the practice falling short of the theory.

Compatibilities: Otters are compatible with Crows (22 September and
22 October), Falcons (21 March – 19 April) and Deer (21 May – 20 June).

11.13 HEALTH

Otter people usually keep in good shape and are keen on health foods and
preventative medicine. Most of their health problems will stem from the

circulatory system and later in life they are likely to be prone to varicose veins and hardening of the arteries.

11.14 AFFINITY COLOUR: **Silver**

Silver is a metallic colour and is the colour of electrical impulse, of lightning, and of the brain. It is a colour that emanates from the mental body and is related to ideas.

Silver is the colour reflected by the Moon, with which it is closely associated for it represents the receptive and creative side of Nature. It indicates the intuitive aspect of the mind which enables one to 'see' beyond the intellect.

Silver turns black unless it is polished and worked on, so silver is representative of the changing side of one's nature and has to be worked on in order for it to be transformed. Silver pulls towards a perfection that lies beyond the understanding.

11.15 ADVANTAGEOUS TIMES

Best months of the year for Otter people are from 20 January to 18 February, from 21 May to 20 June, and from 22 September to 22 October.
Best day of the week is Saturday.
Best times of the day are from 11 a.m. to 1 p.m. and 11 p.m. to 1 a.m.

11.16 OUTWARD (CONSCIOUS) AIM AND INNER (SUBCONSCIOUS) DESIRE

The conscious aim of Otters is to know for themselves. It is knowledge that is not so much acquired as experienced.

The inner desire, however, is for wisdom, which is knowing why and putting that knowledge to work for the benefit of all.

11.17 SPIRITUAL ALCHEMY

The Otter person has an abundance of elemental Air in the spiritual make-up which provides them with a whirlpool of ideas and a mental activity that takes them with exhilaration in all directions.

The stability of Earth and the soothing qualities of Water are needed to provide practical shape for the products of their mind so their ideas can be manifested in physical reality. By studying the Earth Medicine Web, Otters will find examples among the totems of the acquisition and application of Earth and Water energies and should seek to emulate them.

Otter is provided with a negative polarity at directional and cyclical level (– –) and with positive polarity through elemental Air (+ +). The spiritual sexuality is male (+), so the totality is towards the outgoing and thrusting. The combination is thus (– –, + + and +).

11.18 LIFE-CHALLENGES

Otter has to learn the mastery of manifesting what is visualized in the mind.

Otters will be faced with experiences where dreams may be turned into possibilities, and possibilities firmed up into probabilities, and with an outcome in practical reality. But each time it will mean finding the courage to act in accordance with one's inner knowledge.

When Otters find themselves hemmed in and in a rut, they might well bear in mind the motto of the British SAS – 'Who Dares, Wins.'

11.19 PRIMARY FUNCTION AND LIFE-PATH

The primary function of Otter is to reform and invent through discovery.

The life-path is lit by the light of hope for the future. But there is another light – one that is fragile but long-lasting like the light of the stars. It is a light that reveals the oneness of existence and that separation is but an illusion, and that the spiritual 'sky' and the physical 'Earth' are, indeed, woven together. That is the light Otter is being led to see by.

On this path the traveller is led by a guiding vision of the future that is seen to be growing out of the struggles, disappointments, and even catastrophes of the past and present.

The prime purpose is the faith that is the assurance of things to come.

11.20 THE I CHING TRIGRAM: **Sun. The Gentle Wind.**

Those born during the Cleansing Time are on the North position on the Wheel of the Year.

The Gentle Wind implies that which is adaptable, flexible, but persistent. It stresses the need to keep your ideal clearly focused in the mind as you explore thoroughly.

11.21 HOW TO COPE WITH OTTERS

Be direct. Keep to the point. Otters get impatient with wafflers and time-wasters. Say what you mean and mean what you say in dealing with Otters.

The quickest way to get an Otter off your back is to bore them!

Wolf

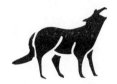

SUMMARY

Birth dates:	19 February – 20 March (22 August – 21 September in the Southern hemisphere).
Earth influence:	The Blustery Winds Time.
Influencing wind:	The North Winds. *Totem:* Buffalo.
Direction:	North-north-east.
Predominant elements:	Water with Air.
Elemental clan:	Frog (Water) Clan.
Birth and animal totem:	Wolf.
Plant totem:	Plantain.
Mineral totem:	Jade.
Polarity totem:	Brown Bear.
Affinity colour:	Blue/green.
Personality:	Compassionate. Benevolent. Generous. Artistic. Gentle.
Feelings:	Deep.
Intention:	Understanding.
Nature:	Trusting.
Positive traits:	Sympathetic. Adaptable. Impressionable. Sensitive.
Negative traits:	Impractical. Vague. Timid. Indecisive.
Sex-drive:	Tender.
Compatibilities:	Woodpeckers, Brown Bears and Snakes.
Conscious aim:	Freedom.
Subconscious desire:	Identity.
Life-path:	Love.
I Ching trigram:	☰ Chi'en. The Creative Heaven. Changing of desire into reality.
Must cultivate:	Intuition. Creativity. Understanding.
Must avoid:	Timidity. Indolence. Impracticality.
Spiritual alchemy:	Yin predominates.
Starting totems:	Wolf. Buffalo. Frog. Plantain. Jade. Brown Bear.

12. Wolf

12.1 BIRTH MONTH: 19 February – 20 March

12.2 EARTH INFLUENCE: The Blustery Winds Time

This third cycle of the North is one that brings rapid changes it is a time of atmospheric turbulence when the winds are blustery, quickly changing their direction. It is a time when warmer temperatures bring the rains that take away the last remnants of the winter snow and ice and refresh the land in preparation for new life that is about to blossom forth.

People born in this time, like the gusty winds, are quick to change direction and possess an ability to direct their energies often in seemingly opposite directions. They have a resilience to recover quickly from disappointment or adversity and to bounce back with equal vigour and determination.

12.3 SOLAR INFLUENCES

This is a time of great anticipation as the Sun moves into the last segment in the yearly cycle. Winter is over, but although the periods of darkness are shortening and the Sun is beginning to wax towards the warmer months, it is not yet spring. It can, perhaps, be described as an 'in-between' time, a period of anticipation and of promise, and that is the essence of the solar influence on those born at this time.

The related Sun sign is Pisces.

12.4 INFLUENCING WIND: North Winds
DIRECTION: North-north-east

The North is the power of purity and renewal and is associated also with wisdom and knowledge, while the East is the power of awakening and of illumination. So the north-north-east is movement from North to East, an 'in-between' area which might be likened to the period after a night's sleep when one is stirring into wakefulness but is not yet fully awake, when the physical body is recharged, refreshed and renewed but the consciousness is closer to the spirit for the human entity is still absorbing the lessons which are sometimes reflected in dream experiences. This knowledge is received inwardly from the spirit during sleep and absorbed for use outwardly in the physical, emotional, and mental activities in the time of wakefulness ahead.

This 'in-between' nature of the north-north-east is indicated in those people born during the Blustery Winds Time by their sensitivity to mystical matters, their psychic potentials, and their refined intuitive sense.

Purification and renewal can be coupled together and understood in the sense of a drawing in of the energy and lessons of past experiences so they can be refined within, before there is a bursting forth once more into new life and new directions in the insatiable drive for knowledge and wisdom.

The totem of the North is the *buffalo*, an animal revered by the American Indians because it gave totally of itself so that man might survive, providing not only meat for food, but material for clothing and the tipi home, and even for utensils and implements. The buffalo symbolized the great sustaining power of the North, and the revived spirit renewed after refreshment and nourishment to explore and experience again without limitation. (See also 10.4).

12.5 INFLUENCING ELEMENTS: Water with Air

Air, as was discussed under the two previous winter seasons, is the element of the mind. Purification, which is stressed so strongly as an essential activity of the North, is thus the activity of clearing the mind. For what reason? So that the will may be focused for creative activity. The purification stressed has nothing to do with sin or any religious sense of morality. It has to do with clearing the mind of the clutter of tensions and anxieties, removing the debris of everyday concerns and frustrations, shifting the weight of tiredness that comes from all the effort of living. It is simply an act of preparing the way for creative mental activity.

Knowledge, too, is emphasized in the North, so what is being stressed here is the discovery of the knowledge of using man's most valuable tool, which is the mind. But in the north-north-east, Air is blended with elemental Water. Water, as was discussed under the three Times of the summer season, has to do with the feelings and emotions, with sentiment and compassion. Just as physical water must contain gaseous air in order to remain fresh, and clouds need to be conveyed to a height where the air is cooled and condensed to fall as rain and nourish the Earth, so elemental Air and elemental Water balance one another in the human experience. In the human experience the intellect (Air) requires the sensitivity of the feelings (Water) so that the thoughts and deeds are tempered with right understanding.

Part of the purpose of life for those born in the Blustery Winds Time is learning to balance these two vital forces so that one is not just drifting along in a cloud of dreams and aspiration, nor being tossed about and sucked into a whirlpool of emotions.

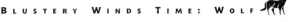

12.6 ELEMENTAL CLAN: Frog (Water) Clan

People whose birthdays fall between 19 February and 20 March are born into the Frog Clan and their association with the Water element imparts to them deep feelings and strong emotions. Indeed, they have the capacity to come into tune with things at all levels because of the intensity of their feelings. However, they need to attain maturity and wisdom to understand and cope with the emotions that surge through them.

Frog Clan people have a great empathy for others and are usually the ones others confide in when they are experiencing difficulties in their emotional lives. Instinctively they feel that somehow Frog Clan people understand them.

Frog Clan people are more sensitive than most of the phases of the Moon. They are still, like calm water, when the Moon is dark, and rippling with emotional energy when the Moon is full.

12.7 BIRTH AND ANIMAL TOTEM: Wolf

The wolf is an ancestor of the domestic dog and a powerful and muscular animal with a broad chest, pointed ears, and a thick, bushy tail. Wolves vary in colour from white in Arctic regions, to grey and through shades of brown to almost black. They are now almost extinct in most of Europe, and even in North America are a threatened species.

Wolves live in mountainous and forest regions and in the Arctic tundra and hunt alone or in pairs or packs. They have an enduring relationship with their mate, and pairs stay together for life.

The wolf was a highly regarded animal among the ancient tribes of northern Europe. It was a totem animal among the ancient Celts and the period just before the arrival of spring was regarded as the Wolf-month in some traditions.

The American Indians associated the wolf with mountains and high places and as a teacher and guide to sacred things. A close relative of the wolf is the coyote – the North American equivalent of the jackal and which was looked upon as the sacred trickster because it used clowning and cunning as part of its strategy. It seemed to offer a justification for tribal shamans to use what we might call showmanship and surprise as part of their 'equipment' and ways of presenting spiritual truths and the extra-ordinary wrapped up in the substance of the ordinary and the everyday.

Wolf people, like their totem animal, are sensitive and intuitive and have a head for heights of both mind and spirit. They share the wolf's need to have its own clearly defined territory whether it is a home, job, or a relationship, and they are upset when intruded upon without invitation. Their intuitiveness is such that they are able to discern quickly the attitudes and intentions of others, however well-hidden these are on the surface.

Wolf people find it difficult to handle their emotions and feel vulnerable if they allow their emotions to flow too freely, though they suffer depression when they are repressed. Because of this dilemma they sometimes have difficulty in reaching decisions over personal relationships. Learning balanced control of the emotions is very much a part of the purpose of life experienced by Wolves.

Like their totem animal, Wolf people look for a permanent relationship. Changing partners can have a devastating effect on the Wolf temperament.

Like the animal, Wolf people are hunters, too, but their 'prey' is in the realm of philosophy and religion, for they seek out and stalk that which may appear to give meaning and purpose to their life.

They, too, have a natural aptitude for presenting unpalatable information in an acceptable form. This ability often makes them good handlers of children, and their manner is such that they can soften the blow of bad news.

12.8 PLANT TOTEM: Plantain

There are many varieties of plantain (*Plantago lanceolate*) which grows in wasteland and fields and on roadsides. Its most common variety has hairy, cylindrical, grooved stems which curve upwards and bear a single head of white flowers around a dense, brownish spike. It has broad, dark-green leaves.

Plantain was renowned among Amerindians for the variety of its healing properties. It was used to dispel mucous congestion, especially catarrh, and for digestive disorders like gastritis and enteritis. Its fresh leaves were used to soothe insect stings and bites, and also for cuts and sores. The oil from the leaves was used as a balm for skin disorders, and the plantain root was used to relieve toothache.

Wolf people, like their plant totem, are versatile, too, in the field of healing. They have a comforting manner and an ability to soothe and to harmonize at both external and internal levels. And like their plant totem, they need to be well-rooted in Earth in order to thrive.

12.9 MINERAL TOTEM: Jade

Jade is a waxy stone composed of sodium aluminium silicate and its colour is usually a soothing green. It is one of the toughest of stones and able to withstand great pressure and this is an indication of one of its outstanding qualities. It was greatly valued by Indians and by ancient peoples and associated with qualities of clarity, wisdom, justice and loyalty.

Jade is associated with peace and tranquillity and with cleansing. It is said to act on the glands affected by the chakras, causing them to dispel impurities. It is also soothing to the nerves. Held in the hand, jade exudes a feeling of warmth and tenderness.

Some Indians used jade in healing by placing the stone on the area of the body affected. They associated it with longevity.

Jade is said to emit soothing vibrations and to dispel negativity. It is, therefore, an important stone to have in one's possession and to have in one's home.

12.10 POLARITY TOTEM: Brown Bear

The flow of spiritual energy with Wolf people inclines them towards philosophical, mystical and religious interests. They are strongly intuitive and have inherent psychic abilities.

It is essential for them to attain and maintain balance by keeping themselves well grounded in practical realities. Brown Bear shows that there need be no conflict between spiritual aspirations and physical attainments. With proper balance it is possible for Wolves to be comfortable in both these realms, and indeed that is part of their life-purpose.

12.11 PERSONALITY EXPRESSION
Adult

Compassionate, benevolent, generous, artistic Wolf. Wolves are warm sympathetic and understanding, and are generally the ones people turn to in times of stress and difficulty because they so readily understand any situation that is brought to their attention. The trouble is that they have a tendency to be affected by the emotional state of the ones they have been talking to or helping, with the result that they often feel drained afterwards. This is because Wolves are like psychic sponges. They need, therefore, to be discriminating because there will be those who will endeavour to draw strength and vitality from them. This may be difficult because Wolves arrive at decisions by feeling rather than by logic or instinct.

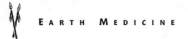

Wolf people need to recognize that they need time on their own periodically to cleanse themselves of the negativity they have absorbed from others and from the environment that they have been in, then they are fresh again to face the demands that are constantly made upon them.

Wolves must have this freedom as well as freedom of movement, of thought and of self-expression. They need to be free to make their own choices rather than have them imposed, otherwise they become inhibited, confused, frustrated and sour. But while they have this urge for freedom themselves, they are often drawn into helping those who are confined or restricted in some way or are victims of ill treatment.

Wolves are regarded as pretty gullible, but this is the result of their desire to want to believe people. They are frequently confronted with the harsher side of life and their trust and genuine concern for others is not always rewarded, especially by the less-evolved souls who can scarcely rise high enough to say 'thank you'. It is therefore essential for the well-being of Wolves that they have opportunities to recuperate and to regain their inner strength, then they will continue to maintain their fluidity and adaptability that is matched by few others.

Over-sensitive to criticism, Wolves find it difficult to stand apart from any work they have done, especially if it is creative endeavour. Any adverse comment or remark, even if it is intended constructively, is often taken as a personal criticism and an attack on Wolf's self-esteem.

Wolf people have a love of beauty whether in Nature or in a work of art, in music, literature, poetry and craftwork – whatever is pleasing to the eye, the ear or the intellect.

Wolf's philosophical attitude to life is expressed in their basic adaptability to any situation or environment in which they find themselves: they simply make the best of it.

Positive traits: Compassionate. Sympathetic. Sensitive. Adaptable. Intuitive. Impressionable. Artistic. Musical.

Negative traits: Indecisive. Vague. Impractical. Timid. Easily confused.

Vocational possibilities: Arts. Astronomy. Astrology. Dancing. Design. Military. Literary work. Law. Social work. Music.

Child

Wolf babies seem to get what they want, not by yelling but by their sweet smiles and winning ways. They seldom throw tantrums and just charm you into capitulation.

The Wolf child needs plenty of attention and at school needs encouragement and assurances about abilities. It needs gentle discipline, otherwise the Wolf child may grow up thinking it can always get what it wants.

Parent

Wolves make fine parents because they understand the needs of individual children and are happy to devote time to them. Above all they respect the dignity of childhood, possibly because they themselves are still children at heart.

The Wolf father enjoys his children as babies and when they are teenagers and have their own point of view, but sometimes finds the school years difficult and prefers to put the main responsibility on to the wife.

Wolf mother can perhaps be over-anxious about the welfare of her offspring and is always aware when they are having some problem or difficulty. She demonstrates her affection for them in many different ways.

12.12 ROMANCE AND SEX

Wolves are romantics and need love and affection more than they need food. When Wolves give their hearts it is for keeps. They are gentle and caring lovers and need a responsive partner for they thrive on the closeness and the sharing that love-making brings.

The female Wolf likes to look pretty. She is soft, sentimental and sensitive and doesn't necessarily always want full-bloodied, raw and passionate sex. She responds to soft words, tender kisses and warm embraces.

The male Wolf will idolize his lover, sometimes to the point that the poor girl finds it difficult to live up to his image of her.

In marriage Wolves will expend more energy on their partner's behalf than on their own and if badly matched can find themselves becoming doormats.

Spiritual sexuality: The spiritual polarity of Wolf is feminine (–).

Compatibilities: Wolves are compatible with Woodpeckers (those born between 21 June and 21 July), Brown Bear (22 August to 21 September) and Snakes (23 October to 22 November).

12.13 HEALTH

Wolf people enjoy their food and have a tendency to become overweight and this can result in circulatory problems, varicose veins and high blood-pressure. They have an above-average interest in natural remedies and alternative medicine, possibly because many have an allergy to certain allopathic drugs or have suffered side-effects from them.

12.14 AFFINITY COLOUR: **Blue/green**

The influencing colour of Wolf people is a combination of blue and green – the colour of the imaginative and discriminating with a deep desire to help others whilst remaining aloof.

Blue is the colour of the sky, which represents the spiritual aspects of life, while green is the colour of Nature and represents the temporal. Blue is the link with the endless cycles of life and with the uplifting spiritual forces, while green is the colour of harmony on the material plane. Blue is the striving for freedom and the love of truth and beauty, while green is the stability of solid foundation. Blue seeks the evolution of the self within the infinity of space, while green seeks growth and development within the limitations of form.

Green is mid-way between the red and violet ends of the spectrum and signifies balance – serenity amid continual change – the balancing of yellow (mind) and blue (spirit). Green wants to nourish and develop, while blue wants to elevate and make infinite. Yellow is the 'hidden' colour in green, and yellow is the intellect and the ability to understand.

So blue-green is the endeavour to nourish and develop that which through life-experiences the individual comes to recognize is of true value and which cannot be transmuted through the Law of Change because it is of infinite and permanent worth. The blue-green ray thus makes the Wolf person discriminating and discerning.

12.15 ADVANTAGEOUS TIMES

Best months of the year for Wolf people are from 19 February to 20 March, 21 June to 21 July, 23 October to 22 November, and 23 November to 21 December.

Best day of the week is Thursday.

Best times of the day are from 1 p.m. to 3 p.m.

12.16 OUTWARD (CONSCIOUS) AIM AND INNER (SUBCONSCIOUS) DESIRE

Wolf's outer (conscious) aim is to break free from entanglements and restrictions and to become detached from limitations imposed in the past.

The inner (subconscious) desire is to reach the source and essence of being in order to obtain cosmic consciousness, which is total freedom.

12.17 SPIRITUAL ALCHEMY

As we have seen, the combination of Air and Water is a necessary balance in order for the primary function of each element to be fulfilled. The abundant activity of Air and the elevation of the aspirations must be balanced with the waters of emotion and by the depth of character. The key is balance.

The directional influence is from cold to cool (– +) and the elemental pull is Air (+) and Water (–). The spiritual sexuality is feminine (–) so the emphasis is on the receptive and nurturing polarity.

The combination is thus (– +, + – and –).

12.18 LIFE-CHALLENGES

Wolves are likely to spend some part of their lives finding and exploring answers to questions of life's meaning and purpose, and are likely to be interested in the possible existence and nature of an afterlife.

The repetitive nature of certain life-experiences, due to the soul's wish to clear away past attachments and confront those lessons still to be learned, should be seen as a challenge to find the point of balance from which true progress can be made.

Must cultivate: Intuition. Creativity. Understanding.

Must avoid: Timidity. Indolence. Procrastination.

12.19 PRIMARY FUNCTION AND LIFE-PATH

The primary function of Wolf is understanding the meaning of love and nurturing it into outward manifestation.

This is the last path on the Wheel of Life, but it is not the end of the road. Rather it is an elusive world where boundaries have dissolved and where new potentials are arising.

It is a path that indicates an unfoldment of deeper latent abilities and which stimulates an urge to bring them to the peak of fulfilment and achievement – to reach for the mountaintops.

The prime purpose of this path is to bring about a realization that there

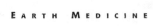

are no endings and no beginnings – only changes – as the traveller rides the spirals of eternity, and that what is of true value has its potential in love, is fashioned in love, and finds its fulfilment in love.

12.20 THE I CHING TRIGRAM: Chi'en. The Creative Heaven.

People born during the Blustery Winds Time are positioned on the north-north-east on the Wheel of the Year.

The Creative Heaven indicates that the emotionalism of an idea is what changes desire into reality.

12.21 HOW TO COPE WITH WOLVES

Wolves respond to love, kindness and consideration. They have an instinctive reaction, so never betray their confidence or you will lose their trust.

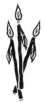

The Practice

Wakan-Tanka's Talk

Wakan-Tanka talks with me
Through the pages of no book
Penned by the thoughts of men.
No words, no creed, no dogma
Writes He to bind me to a clan.
In flight of birds that wing their way
To lands beyond my sight
In trees that root and take their time
To grow to their full height
In flowers whose petals hold
Such fragrance in their clasp
And every single animal
With purpose in its grasp
In Sun that rises with each Dawn
To herald a new start
In Moon that holds the ebb and flow
Of tides within Her hand
In Venus, Jupiter and Mars
And stars that form His heavenly band
In everything that breathes
And moves
And crawls
And flows
And stands
Wakan-Tanka talks with me.

Kenneth Meadows, 1988

The Path to Rediscovery

S ELF-IMPROVEMENT IS NOT ABOUT BETTERING THE SOCIAL IMAGE or gaining the approval of others. It is getting rid of what is inhibiting us from becoming what we want to be – a reflection of our True Self. How do we find – or rather, rediscover – our True Self, our own, individual Higher Self? Our Soul Self?

The American Indians, like the ancients, approached life in accordance with the principle, 'As Within, So Without'. It was a principle based upon the premise that the external world that was being perceived was the substance of spirit.

Space – that immeasurable quality that appears between objects in the external world and in which all living things live and move and have their being – was regarded as the substance of eternity, which was a condition of universal Spirit. Every human being occupied space in the external world and a place in eternity because the human being was an individualization of a universal Spirit.

But space is *in* all things, impregnating everything, and existing in all things. As modern science has discovered, all matter is composed largely of 'empty' space. Nothing is actually 'solid' at all, although it may *appear* so. Every tiny atom, with its electrons whirling at tremendous speeds around the neutron, is like an infinitesimal solar system and, like the universe, is mostly space. So vast is this 'emptiness' of space within the atom that the neutron might be likened to a pea in the whistle of a referee standing on the centre spot in the middle of a huge sports stadium, with the electrons, even smaller than the pea, following an orbit beyond the outside of the stands.

So there is space within as well as space that can be perceived without. The external world was regarded as containing the substance of Spirit and the internal world as containing the essence of Spirit before it comes into existence as substance. Since there was only one universal Spirit – humanity, and the animal, plant and mineral 'kingdoms' were all manifestations of that one great Spirit.

That was the essence of the spirituality of the Amerindian and of all ancient peoples. When we grasp that concept we can perhaps begin to understand why the Amerindian enjoyed a relationship with Earth and with Nature that extended far beyond the protectiveness of today's conservationist, the concern of the ecologist, and even the sincerity of the naturalist. It was a communion with Nature that recognized, with all the love and simplicity and innocence of a child whose trust and understanding had not yet been impaired by the complexities and cynicisms of adulthood's sophisticated knowledge, that Nature was not something that was *separate* from themselves but, in a sense, an extension. Nature, with all its wonders and beauties, was a manifestation of that one universal mind in which the individual human entity and all of Creation was immersed. Each human being was thus an individuation within that one great Spirit.

American Indians of old had no concept of the human mind. What could be seen, heard, touched, tasted and smelled was physical, and what could not be seen, heard, touched, tasted or smelled was non-physical and therefore perceived as being spiritual. What we call the mind is also intangible and similarly cannot be measured, weighed or dissected as can anything material. The mind might be regarded as an aspect of the spirit for it is related to intelligence. What some American Indians referred to as Great Spirit might, in the terminology of present-day psychology, be referred to as Universal Mind.

Within each human being was a non-physical inner reality which in modern psychological terms is referred to as the psyche. 'Psyche' is a Greek word which actually means 'soul' and 'breath'. The psyche, or soul, is thus likened to breath. The breath of life is an inbreathing and an outbreathing – a pulsation of that living soul.

But if the psyche or soul is non-physical, how does it breathe? It undergoes its inbreathing by drawing in energies from the impressions and experiences of the outward, conscious activity in the external world of physical reality. Its outbreathing is the outgoing energies of the psyche's inner activity into the external world. So the way the external world is perceived is, to an extent, conditioned by the inner world of which we are not normally consciously aware. This Looking Out and Looking In is another movement of the yang and yin, then This and That, in each of us. Yang is the Conscious Without, the apparent external world of physical appearances. Yin is the Unconscious Within, the invisible reality.

The psyche, or soul, is a means by which the human being perceives. It is not the originator of thought. It is not the self. It is an instrument or vehicle of thought and it operates on different levels of awareness.

Level 1: is the conscious, and is the middle realm or Middle World.

Level 2: is the subconscious, and is the lower realm or Underworld.

Level 3: is the unconscious and it, too, is in the lower realm and deeper still in the Underworld.

Level 4: is the superconscious and is in the upper realm or Higher World and is the realm of pure essence or spirit.

Level 1 might be regarded as the level of awareness of the physical world of 'ordinary' reality. It is our concept of what is happening to us and all around us and which we consider as 'real'.

Level 2 might be regarded as the level of imagination and instinct, and of symbols and images. It is part of the world we might regard as 'non-ordinary' reality. It is the subconscious. It is the place of 'becoming'.

Level 3 is deeper still. It is the area of unconscious activity which keeps our heart beating regularly, that controls our breathing and bodily functions of which we are totally unaware. It is the level of automatism.

Level 4 is the superconscious which is beyond all these states. It is the level of dreamlike being. It is the level of our true reality, our spirit self.

We spend most of our time on Level 1 which is the level that engages our physical senses. If we liken the mind to a globe or, perhaps, an onion, the conscious level is like the surface which can be peeled away. We might call this level the surface mind. Beneath it is another level – which psychology calls the subconscious mind. It is a lower mind, an almost robotic mind since it acts on instructions that penetrate through to it. Deeper still, if we peel away the subconscious, is the unconscious mind, the automatic mind that carries out the work.

Then there is the inner mind, the mind of our own inner reality which is at the very core of our being. It is the superconscious mind, the mind of the 'divinity' within which some have called the 'soul' within everyone. It is the essence of our true identity and of our Higher Self. It is our superconscious – our soul or 'spirit' self. It is part of the world of unreal reality where time and space laws do not apply, where all that ever was, is now, and ever will be, has noumenal existence.

Let us always remember that through that part of our consciousness called imagination, we can actually create – we can change reality. In a very real sense, then, the Great Spirit is in us, as in all, and we can channel Its creative power.

Mankind knew nothing of the subconscious mind or the so-called superconscious until the end of the nineteenth century yet the American Indian shaman and the shamans of Europe and other cultures had a knowledge of their existence that went back thousands of years. Of course, they did not identify them by such names, but personified them. None the less, they were aware of their existence, function and abilities.

The shaman considered that a human being was composed of four 'selves'. There was the self concerned with normal, everyday, conscious activity and which functioned in the realm of physical reality. This was the 'middle' self functioning in the realm of 'appearances' which some American Indians referred to as the 'Tonal' world and the European shaman called the 'Middle World'. It is the realm of what I have previously described as the Surface Mind.

The Middle 'self' operated in partnership with the Low 'self' which corresponded with the concept of the subconscious of modern psychology. The Low 'self' was the seat of conscience which was conditioned by concepts of right and wrong, morality and immorality, impressed into it through the Middle 'self'. Whereas the Middle 'self' was reasoning, the Low 'self' was unreasoning and acted on instructions which filtered through to it.

The Low 'self' was sometimes referred to as 'the Child Self' – the 'child' that is within us whatever our age and position in life and which finds expression in our actions when we act 'like a child'.

According to the ancient teaching, the Low 'self' relayed thought-patterns to the Higher Self with which it was said to be linked by an invisible cord. The Higher Self was the Soul Self, the True Self that had permanence and functioned on a level that was above that of normal consciousness and in a state of timelessness which the shaman called the Nagual. The Higher Self was the protector and guardian of the Middle 'self' and the Low 'self' through which it was enabled to experience material existence.

The Higher Self also fashioned the thought-patterns fed to it from the Low 'self' into thought forms that materialized as the Middle 'self's' conscious reality in the future. The thought-patterns were energized by the vital prana or mana force which I referred to in Chapter 6. The strength and power of this pranic or manic energy determined the clarity of the thought-pattern from the Low 'self' and thus the actuality of the thought-form and its ultimate materialization. This vital force responded to mind.

There was also a Body 'self' which was the centre of consciousness of the physical body. The Body 'self' is that part of you that acts instinctively in times of crisis, and that is mostly concerned with physical survival and the desire to perpetuate itself. It is that part of you that 'fights' or 'flees' when threatened.

All four 'selves' are part of your totality. The Higher Self might be regarded as the eternal, spiritual self; the Middle 'self' as the temporary personality of this present life – your everyday self; the Low 'self' is the 'child' within, and the Body 'self' is that part of you whose emphasis is on the physical, on self-preservation and survival and self-interest. The Higher Self has eternal life but seeks experience whereas the Body 'self' at the other end of the polarity has experience and seeks eternal life.

This concept of the four 'selves' and four 'minds' was a key to the magik of the shamans and of their healing powers. It was also a key to the question of human identity. Each of us, at some time, has questioned the truth of our own identity that goes beyond the name we were given at birth or acquired on marriage. The eternal questions of human existence have crossed our minds and we have sought answers to them. But the answers seem to elude even the most educated minds. Philosophers have tried: they offer us hope. Religionists have tried: they offer us faith. Spiritualists have tried: they offer us comfort. But none give us the answers we seek.

We expect the answers to come from someone in 'authority', from someone who is 'qualified' and better educated than ourselves; from someone more spiritually 'advanced' perhaps – from a spiritual teacher, a philosopher, a religious leader, a mystic, a guru; someone in the 'know'. We never think to look within. We never turn to the one absolute authority in our own lives, the one who really knows us better than anyone, the one who was with us at our birth, is our constant companion throughout every moment of every day and will there at our death: our 'Real' Self; our 'True' Self – our Higher Self. The Soul Self that is to be found in the one place we have never looked – within. We have looked everywhere but within.

The Higher Self is not somewhere 'up *there*' above us, not in some inaccessible 'heavenly' realm in Outer Space, but 'in' *here*, deep 'inside' us in 'Inner' Space, but existing on a higher vibratory rate than our conscious, everyday 'self'.

We have each of us been so conditioned by parents, by the educational system, by our cultural background, and by society in which we live, to look outwards for knowledge as if it were a commodity that came from beyond ourselves that we much feed on and absorb. But what we obtain in this way is only external knowledge – knowledge that comes by and through the Surface Mind, knowledge that is based on appearances, on experimentation, on arguments, judgements, opinions and beliefs. We are not told that we can have access to an inner knowledge – a knowledge that comes from within and is based on realities that exist beyond the appearances of physical existence. We are not told because the way to that knowledge has become lost, or hidden or obscured.

Our Surface Mind has been thus programmed by other people – first by our parents, then our teachers, and by the traditions and customs of the society in which we were born. Its input has been the beliefs and attitudes, opinions and prejudices and influences of others. It has been conditioned by the consumer society in which we live, by advertisers who stimulate desire. It is manipulated by the media, by politicians, by commentators, analysts and instant pundits. It is fashioned by husband, wife or lover, by parents, by friends and neighbours, by people we work with or work for. The Surface Mind causes us to act as others expect us to act. It causes us to believe what others say about us. It causes us to conform to the image others have of us. We can rarely be ourselves.

With all the constant chatter and incessant sound which engulfs us from the world around, we never pause long enough to listen for the answers about ourselves which can come only from within. Yet only the 'You' within knows you intimately enough to know who You are, what you're doing here, and where you're supposed to be heading. That 'You' has known the answers all along. The trouble is that the 'little' you, the you of the Surface Mind, has cut itself off from the recall channel and has lost its way.

If you truly want the answers, you must have the courage to take off the 'headset' that allows you to be under such constant bombardment. You have to learn to listen to the Internal Mind that will help you to know the truth about yourself and bring you the contentment that you crave. And what is contentment? Contentment is when you are not aware of actually wanting anything. Of being satisfied with what the moment holds and drawing pleasure and profit from the time you are in. Just imagine – finding pleasure and knowledge in the moment! That might seem an impossible dream, but you can attain it if you will because, essentially, that is an overall purpose of life.

Life is intended to be pleasurable, not something to put up with, to be suffered and endured. Life is wonder-ful. Life is purpose-ful. Life is for the purpose of gaining knowledge through the wonder of experience. That knowledge has little to do with the gathering of useless facts which sometimes masquerades as 'education': it is the knowledge that can be transformed into wisdom so that wisdom can be activated into Love. That is the essence of the message of all true religion, which is man's approach to the sublime. Light, law and love – the sacred expressions of the 'mind' of the Great Spirit.

That is how we 'evolve'. For the true purpose of the 'evolutionary' process is the cultivation of the Spirit. That is what it is all about.

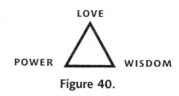

Figure 40.

Part Three of this book is intended to provide a finer tuning of Earth Medicine and to indicate practical uses of its principles. We make use of them and experience for ourselves their validity by developing a capacity to align with the universal mind and by coming into harmony with its manifestations. Once we begin to do this, we extend and expand our conscious awareness and develop a perception of that which is beyond 'ordinary' reality, thus cultivating the spirit.

We make a start by becoming aware of the cycles of activity within Nature, which is demonstrating to us how the universal mind operates, and then by putting ourselves into harmony with it.

Consider that nothing can be done without love, wisdom and power, and that they form a triangle that must be balanced (see Figure 40). Even to make a cup of coffee requires all three – the love or desire to will the act, the wisdom to know how to do it, and the power to complete it. These are the three attributes of the Spirit which are being cultivated, and to ensure that we do not get it wrong and ourselves out of balance, we learn from aligning ourselves with Nature. Power without wisdom and love is dangerous. Wisdom without power and love is dry and academic. Love without power and wisdom is weak and foolish.

The Medicine Wheel teachings inherent in this system of Earth Medicine help us to relate consciously to our own individual Spirit so that the life we are living comes more into harmony with it. The Higher Self can 'converse' with us in our inner thinking. That is why periods of meditation are so essential – times when we can turn off the chatter of the external world all around us and which wants to consume us so we can 'listen' in the stillness of our own being.

That contact comes to us not through the Surface Mind, the reasoning mind, but intuitively and it comes unexpectedly like a flash of lightning. It is usually followed by a response from the reasoning intellect which will argue against whatever is intuited and then that flash of inspiration becomes lost or at best obscured.

We need to learn to trust our intuitiveness and act upon it, then new courses of action open up before us and our lives come more into harmony with their intended purpose and with the flow of Nature.

'As Within, So Without'

THE PRINCIPLE 'AS WITHIN, SO WITHOUT' BROUGHT WITH IT A recognition by the Amerindians and ancient peoples that what was happening in the natural cycle of activity in the external world of physical reality was a reflection of that within the human entity, and vice versa.

The Circle could be seen as a Wheel of the Year that is constantly turning as the seasons change and the periods of daylight and darkness vary in length, revealing the ebb and flow of time-energy. The gradual unfoldment of the seasons of the year, cycle by cycle, from spring to summer, through autumn and winter, and on again to spring, together with the ebb and flow of the tides of the Moon, were indicative of the way the subtle energies within the human organism operated. It was by coming into harmony with the flow of Nature that a person was able to attain equilibrium between the physical, emotional, mental, sexual and spiritual aspects of their own nature.

Just as the flow of the seasons and the tides of the Moon take place whether we live in a rural area and are sensitive to their moods and changes, or whether we live or work in the concrete surroundings of a big city and are not aware of them, so there is movement of the subtle forces within us whether we are aware of them or not.

I would draw attention to four occasions within the seasonal cycle which indicate specific points of change in the energy potential of Nature and thus within ourselves. These four occasions can be located on the Earth Web and provide co-ordinates by which Time and Space can by synchronized. These four locations are the Winter and Summer Solstices and the Spring and Autumn Equinoxes, each of which is determined by the movement of the Earth around the Sun and the angle of the Earth's surface in relation to the Sun. They are, therefore, solar-orientated.

In pre-Christian Britain (then known as Prydain – Enchanted Isles) and northern Europe, these four turning-points of the yearly cycle were recognized as solar festivals – Ostara (Easter) on the first day of spring (21–24 March), Litha or Midsummer's Day (21–23 June), Mabon on the first day of autumn (21–23 September), and Yule – which later became Christmas – on 21–23 December. The festival dates varied from year to year, but for the purpose of providing an uncomplicated and *practical* working model, mean dates have been selected here. These are 21 March, 21 June, 22 September and 22 December.

The solstices are pivotal points in the year and are when the days are longest or shortest. They are like switches which bring about a change either to increasing light or to decreasing light – from longer nights to longer days, or from shorter days to shorter nights. Each solstice is a pause between a change in Nature. And each provides a vital clue for humans, too, for they are appropriate times to pause and to take stock of your life and to seek to come into harmony with the changing flow of natural forces.

Christmas has its 'festival' origins in ancient times with the celebration of the Winter Solstice (Yule) around 22 December. It was a festival of reunion, of recognizing the importance of one's 'togetherness', with a family and of relationships with other individuals. It was a time to be thankful for family ties and the value of friendships.

The Summer Solstice, on the other hand, around 21 June, was an occasion to celebrate one's individuality and creativity. It was a time to concentrate on *personal* considerations.

Since the solstices are 'switch-over' points in the flow of cosmic and solar energies, they were recognized as opportune times to bring to completion what had gone before in one's personal life, and for fixing the intentions for what one aimed to achieve in the period ahead.

Mid-way between the solstices are the equinoxes, when the days and nights are of equal length. They indicate periods of rapid change in the yearly cycle when the change in the direction of solar and cosmic energies has become plain and noticeable. They emphasize the principle that energy takes time to come into form and to move out of form. The Spring Equinox is the first day of spring (around 21 March) when the increase in light is becoming evident. The Autumn Equinox (around 22 September) is when the waning of the light is becoming apparent.

There were four other periods which were marked in ancient times by festivals which enabled people to identify readily with the energies of Nature and to harmonize with the powers of Nature that were finding expression in the environment around them. These were fire festivals that were associated not with solar but with lunar energies. These Moon festivals were Imbolc

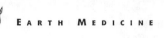

around February eve, Beltain on May eve, Lammas around August eve, and Samhain on November eve.

Because witches also celebrated these festivals and called them Witches' Sabbats, they became associated with witchcraft, but they do not have their origins in witchcraft. Witches were eclectics and borrowed them from one or more ancient sources of origin. Modern witches have devised their own ritualistic and religious interpretations of the meaning of these ancient festivals.

In some divisions of the Christian faith, these very same ancient festivals appear, but they are called 'Saints' Days'.

In each case the symbology has been changed, and in each case has tended to obscure their original relevance.

In ancient Britain and northern Europe people met together on these festival occasions not just to celebrate an annual event in the seasonal cycle, but to become personally and collectively in harmony with the flow of Nature's energies at these pivotal points. Marking these occasions enabled people to *become attuned to Time*. That was their true purpose. By becoming actively involved with the natural forces, they were able to find a focus for their own energies and to bring into being the things that would enhance and enrich their lives, both individually and as members of a family or community.

That was the true purpose of the festivals then, and that purpose is no less sound today whether they are observed by groups of people or merely tapped into by lone individuals recognizing these high points of the year on their own.

Let us now follow the ebb and flow of these tides of Nature through the seasons, and the eight festival occasions of ancient times, because they can help us to understand the cycles of energies within ourselves.

SPRING   *The Tide of Activation*

The Spring Equinox around 21 March marks the balance-point or centre of the time when the life-force rises around the time of Imbolc and the Earth and Nature 'come alive'. The sap rises and shoots appear above the ground and we, too, feel motivated to get things moving again in our lives after the limitations of winter. The influence of the Tide of Activation is not only in Nature around us but also within ourselves.

This tidal power reaches its peak around Beltain (May Eve).

Beltain stresses the unity of the male and female, the pollination aspect of Nature which creates joy and beauty and new life. In our own lives it emphasizes the need for freedom to develop our own potentials and our own individuality.

The Summer Solstice marks the balance-point, or centre, of the time when this Tide of Activation is ebbing and becomes quiescent at Lammas, going 'within' through the Autumn Equinox and Yule (see Figure 41).

This period when the tide of the cosmic energy is running in the Earth is an appropriate time to put the emphasis in one's life on earthly and material things. It is the time to initiate new projects and to develop plans that will bring material benefits to the physical self.

The Tide of Activation is positive and yin moving to yang.

SUMMER *The Tide of Growth*

Summer is the season of rampant growth and rapid progress. The Summer Solstice around 21 June marks the centre or mid-point of the waxing of the Binding Force, the force of molecular attraction, and the Tide of Growth which rose at Beltain and reaches its peak at Lammas on 1 August when creative self-expression reaches its climax.

The Tide of Growth makes us pause to celebrate our own individuality, and take cognisance of our personal attitudes and approaches to life so that we can better focus and consolidate our efforts and make the fullest use of our potentials.

It reaches its peak at the time when the Earth is at its most bounteous and gives so generously of her substance, so it is an appropriate time for us, too, to experience the joy of giving and the gratitude that should come from receiving. The emphasis, then, is on generosity and benevolence.

It is a time also for gathering in the fruits of past efforts, and to experience enjoyment from them. The benefits are not solely materialistic for there is much to be learned from the lessons of past endeavours.

The autumn Equinox marks the balance-point or centre of the time when the Tide of Growth is ebbing and it becomes quiescent at Samhain around 31 October.

The Tide of Growth is also positive and yang.

AUTUMN *The Tide of Recession*

The life-force in Nature goes inwards at Lammas and can be clearly seen to be receding at the Autumn Equinox around 22 September, which is the centre or balance-point in the fall of the Tide of Recession. At Samhain on 31 October the tide has receded to a point when the energies are disappearing into the realm of the unmanifest, so the human emphasis at this time should be on spiritual principles rather than on material benefits. At the human level the pull is to relate more to others and for the support which comes from association with a group, family or community. Samhain indicates the death of the old and the promise of new beginnings and of rebirth. It is a time of transformation and the

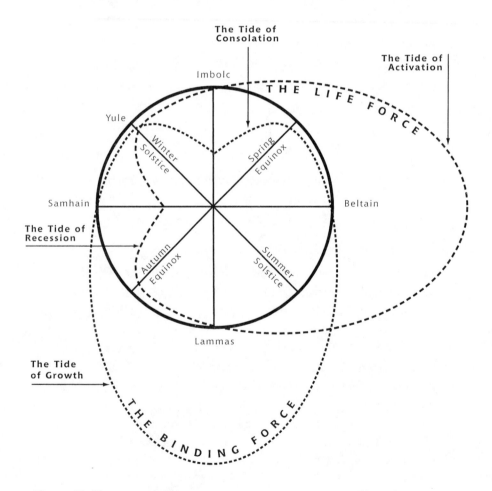

Figure 41. The seasonal tides

change of emphasis from outer activity to inner growth.

Yule at the Winter Solstice marks the balance-point of the life-force in its resurrection path towards Imbolc where it again becomes external.

The Tide of Recession is negative and yang moving to yin.

WINTER   *The Tide of Consolidation*

Winter is the season of withdrawal and consolidation, beginning at Samhain when the Binding Force goes inwards. At the Winter Solstice around 22 December, the tide has reached the mid-point in its passage within to Imbolc where it vanishes into the darkness of the invisible and can no longer be seen or sensed. It is like the darkness of night at the New Moon when the two luminaries, the Sun and the Moon, are no longer visible, but we know they are still 'there', not through any leap of faith, but through the assurance and certainty of true knowledge.

Yule recognizes the importance of sharing, and stresses the value of obligation and responsibility. It celebrates the joy of belonging, and the value of family ties and close relationships, and of goodwill towards all humanity.

Imbolc, celebrated around 2 February, marks the time of making adjustments and of purifying the intent in preparation for the arrival of spring and the transition to a new cycle of activity as the Wheel of the Year turns again. The name implied 'quickening'.

Imbolc brings the first light of illumination. It is like the narrowest crescent of the Moon on a crisp night. Its emphasis is purification, not so much moralistically but in the sense of concentrating and focusing the intentions. It is an excellent time for meditation and contemplation.

The Spring Equinox marks the mid-point in the resurrection path of the Binding Force towards Beltain where it goes external.

The Tide of Consolidation is negative and yin.

Synchronizing with these natural tides of time-energy enables us to put ourselves in harmony with Earth and the life-systems it supports, and to open up channels within ourselves that have become blocked. It leads the

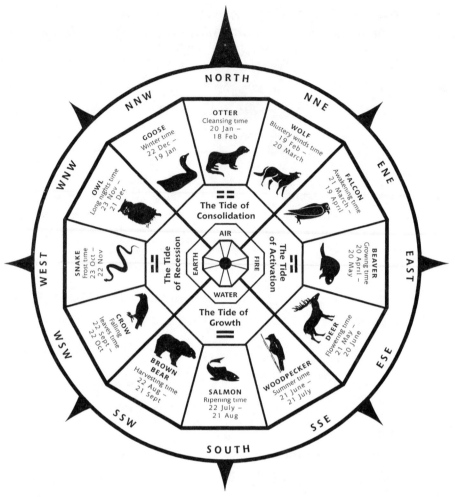

Figure 42. The tides of time-energy on the Earth Web

way to living our lives more purposefully and effectively and to the attainment of the contentment and fulfilment which eludes so much of humanity because it is out of tune with Nature and with the Creation.

Putting ourselves in tune with Nature and with Earth attunes us also to our own Higher Self.

The Personality Mask

WHEN AN AMERINDIAN PAINTED HIS FACE, IT WAS GENERALLY for the purpose of expressing personality, or a particular quality or trait or emotion. Often it was representative of an animal or bird that emphasizes the desired quality or trait. It was a mask – a means of expression.

Likewise, your personality is only an *expression* of you. It is not actually you, any more than your physical body is you. It belongs to you, like the physical body belongs to you. It is yours, but it is not you. It is the way you experience and respond to the world.

The personality 'mask' is what the True Self – the inner 'You' – puts on to perceive the physical world in the dimension of time. According to the oral teachings, there are twelve categories of such 'masks', twelve principal areas of perception, twelve broad ways of expression – one for each segment of the Wheel of the Year. These were examined in some detail in Part Two of this book.

The 'Personality' Self is in conscious existence – a state in which you see, feel, touch, taste, smell, know and think, but are limited by space and time. But the True Self – the inner you – is in a state that is beyond time and space.

Those statements may appear to be either profound sense or simplistic nonsense. Actually they are neither. They are facts of our daily experience. For instance, when you go to sleep you withdraw from conscious existence by leaving the world of the senses. When you wake in the morning you may remark that you had a good night's sleep by not recalling anything of what happened during the sleeping state. You have no memory of that state when you were withdrawn from conscious existence, only an awareness that somehow it was 'good'. During those hours you never ceased to 'be' even though you were not conscious of self.

A lifetime is like the waking time. Death is like the sleep time when we are withdrawn from waking existence yet never cease to 'be'. So each lifetime is like a new 'day' – another opportunity to develop character, which is a condition or quality of the nature of the developing True Self, that inner you. Each lifetime is a challenge to grasp the potentials with which we have each been entrusted, and to nurture the inherent talents into expression and form. Each lifetime is based on the achievements and failures of our former lives. Just as each new day is affected by what has been done in the days before, so our next lifetime will be shaped and conditioned by what we make of the present one. We are what we have become through what we were before.

Your True Self – the inner you – did not come into being on the day of your birth. Only our logical and 'conditioned' thinking leads us to assume there was a 'beginning'. After all, when was the beginning of you? Was it at the time of your birth? Hardly. For did you not exist in your mother's womb before the day of your birth? Perhaps it was the time of your conception? But, surely, that was only when the physical body you occupy began to be knitted together and fashioned in accordance with the DNA code contained within the genes? That was not you, it was only a blueprint for the vehicle being provided for you to occupy for the span of a few years in time. It was only an expression of you. The *real* you, then, has no *material* existence! The personality 'mask' you put on has only temporary existence.

You appeared in the physical world, apparently out of nowhere, and one day you will disappear from the physical world at death and the real you will return from whence it came.

The dimension of existence in which you now appear is the dimension of time. And the timing of your *physical* appearance not only determined the perception point from which you were to look out and observe physical existence, but also the category of personality mask you were to put on and through which to formulate and express your True Self and the Earth influences with which you were to work.

Ancient knowledge postulated twelve broad personality categories, twelve perception positions on the Wheel of the Year, twelve expressions of Earth influences. No position is better or more important than another. Just different. Each provides essential qualities to further the progress and development of the individual True Self behind the personality. No position is more advantageous than another, none easier or more difficult. Each provides responsibilities and challenges, advantages to work with, and disadvantages to overcome. Each contains its own strengths and weaknesses – strengths to enable growth and development, and weaknesses to be turned into strengths.

The Wheel or Web was not regarded as a ring or band which contained these categories in a restrictive way. Form and formlessness, matter and spirit, birth and death, mortality and immortality, time and eternity – all were within this Circle which was itself spiralling out in all directions and in all dimensions. In was in a state of constant motion, but not like a piece of machinery which goes round and round in a repetitive movement. It was a slice of a spiral. One revolution of the spiral brought us back facing the same direction in which we started, but not to the same place because we had moved on and upwards.

In Nature, the Wheel of the Year 'turns' as it is affected by the Sun, which governs the seasons and the days, and by the Moon by which the months and the weeks were once marked. In other words, the Sun and Moon are vital components in the technology of time, which is the dimension we're now in.

The Sun and Moon were also regarded among ancient peoples as representative of the duality of the masculine and feminine principles inherent in Nature, and of the active and passive, conceptual and receptive forces that permeate it.

The Moon, in its feminine aspect, was often represented as presenting the *four* faces of a woman. The Waxing Moon was represented as the face of a young maiden, the Full Moon that of a mother, the Waning Moon that of a grandmother, and the Dark unseen Moon that of an old woman. Each indicated the way energies were being reflected in the world of form on Earth. The Dark 'face' of the Moon was seen as the potential that was hidden and waiting to come into expression, the Waxing Moon as that which was developing and coming into maturity, the Full Moon as the fully developed and mature, the Waning Moon as the giving out and sharing of that which had been nurtured and developed, and back again to the Dark Moon and a period of resting and renewal and absorption before the cycle begins again.

As light from the Moon was seen as being reflected in this cyclical way, so similarly the characteristics of each personality 'mask' were observed to find expression and to develop in four ways, though each was not separate but merged or flowed into the others.

Although the Moon's energies acted on the Earth and on ourselves, the Earth Influences were characterized by the Sun and Earth as well as the Moon. It was not the Moon that was said to govern these influences and responses. The Moon was an *indicator* of the manner of their movement and of their unfolding. The Moon indicated the way these Earth influences were operating.

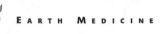

 For instance, the Waxing Moon was seen as a beautiful maiden absorbed in her own attractiveness and drawing things towards her and so was indicative of the *developing* personality.

 The Full Moon was seen as the young mother devoted to her offspring and product of her involvement, and therefore symbolic of the *developed* and mature personality.

 The Waning Moon was represented as the grandmother concerned with the well-being of an entire family community and recognizing the responsibility of giving and sharing what has been learned from the experience of development. It symbolized the *extrovert* personality.

 The Dark face of the Moon, as an old woman, is the least understood and often ignored or even excluded from some Western esoteric teachings. It was both at the 'end' and at the 'beginning' of a cycle and indicated a turning inward, an absorption of what had gone before, and a nurturing of the potential of what was yet to become. In indicated the *introverted* personality. It was symbolic of a concentration of essentials and the banishing of worldly cares.

Broadly speaking, the qualities and characteristics of each personality category and each Earth influence unfold like the petals of a flower. The *developing* personality is like a bud which grips the qualities tightly to itself and is concerned with how everything is affecting it personally, but which is gradually learning to open up. The *developed* personality is one that has brought the qualities to full expression. The *extroverted* personality is one that has developed a more holistic attitude and has learned not only to balance individual needs with those of others, but is outgoing in the desire to share. The *introverted* personality is one that is expressing characteristics with a more spiritual emphasis and with regard to the well-being of the greater whole.

As a general guide, here is a brief summary of the four aspects of each birth totem:

Falcons

The developing Falcon will be full of grandiose schemes, but may lack the staying power to see them through.

The developed Falcon will be generous and good-natured and influence others by example.

The extroverted Falcon is likely to be involved in actions that are mutually beneficial but has a tendency to squander opportunities.

Introverted Falcons will be self-centred and emphasize the need for self-gratification. They are likely to put their own needs first and foremost.

Beavers

Developing Beavers are constructive, but cautious and conventional. They work hard at preparing things for completion.

Developed Beavers are practical and productive, and generous and understanding towards those who share their affections. They have a strong sense of loyalty, and a courage and composure that makes them good companions to have around, especially in times of crisis or danger.

Extroverted Beavers are warm and hospitable, but mentally conservative. They want to rest on their laurels and may resist change. They can be rather apathetic and lethargic.

Introverted Beavers can be obstinate and inflexible. They are mercenary in all things, and seek material reward for everything they do.

Deer

 Developing Deer are adaptable and enjoy variety and plenty of activity. Their sense of curiosity urges them to explore ideas, situations and relationships, but they will generally flee from those which may threaten to tie them down.

 Developed Deer are cheerful, intelligent, versatile and clear-thinking.

 Extroverted Deer are candid and friendly and enjoy exchanging opinions. They are, however, likely to dissipate their energies in directions that are unlikely to be productive and beneficial.

 Introverted Deer are inconsiderate and often lazy. They are easily bored and fickle, susceptible to every influence that comes their way. They tend to lack real purpose.

Woodpeckers

 The developing Woodpecker, though protective and defensive, is usually affable and kindly, and has a ready sympathy towards the needs of others.

 The developed Woodpecker is full of good intentions and the tendency is to want to keep things together. Developed Woodpeckers are persistent and resourceful.

 Extroverted Woodpeckers tend to swing between the extremes of being kindly and considerate on the one hand, and harsh and even bitter on the other.

 Introverted Woodpeckers are self-protecting and hypersensitive. They can be unyielding and unforgiving, and affected by fears and anxieties, most of which are imaginary.

Salmon

22 JULY – 21 AUGUST

 Developing Salmon are virile and versatile and full of go-getting drive, but they need constant praise and encouragement in order to achieve.

 The developed Salmon exudes and inspires confidence. Their cheerfulness and warm-hearted generosity make them good to have around.

 Extroverted Salmon are extravagant and egotistical and easily depressed when things don't go as they want.

 Introverted Salmon can be erratic and impulsive and work themselves into a fury which can be quite destructive.

Brown Bears

22 AUGUST – 21 SEPTEMBER

 Developing Brown Bears are helpful but unassuming, and compassionate without sentimentality.

 Developed Brown Bears are compassionate and understanding with an ability to see things from all angles.

 Extroverted Brown Bears are unselfish and reliable and give strength to others.

 Introverted Brown Bears are fussy and critical and see only the flaws of a situation.

22 SEPTEMBER – 22 OCTOBER

Crows

 Developing Crows are more self-assertive and have a capacity for leadership. They have a gregarious manner.

 Developed Crows are psychologically well-balanced and have few inhibitions. They have a strong sense of impartiality and inspire confidence in those they are with.

 Extroverted Crows will so almost anything to please. Socially, they are good mixers and great conversationalists, and will fall in with the mood of whatever company they're in.

 Introverted Crows are often superficial, indolent and dependent on others.

---

23 OCTOBER – 22 NOVEMBER

Snakes

 Developing Snakes are enterprising and energetic, but impatient. They are not content with half measures, and although intense are prone to make sudden and unexpected changes.

 Developed Snakes are benevolent, deeply philosophical, and absorbed with the mysteries of life. They are passionate about their beliefs and put themselves wholeheartedly into their actions.

 Extroverted Snakes will go out of their way to help others. In their relationships and associations they often bring out the abilities of others.

Introverted Snakes are secretive and aloof. They can be scheming and manipulative. They have an argumentative disposition.

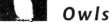

Owls

 Developing Owls are adventurous and constantly on the look-out for opportunities to improve the quality of their lives, but they do have a tendency to be easily side-tracked.

 Developed Owls have a strong sense of justice and an urge to champion individual freedom of expression and action. They have a capacity to balance their idealism with practicality.

 Extroverted Owls can be rather Utopian and extreme in their ideals and rather dogmatic about their beliefs and aspirations. They are prone to be carried away into fanaticism.

 Introverted Owls might be described as essentially moralistic humanists. They tend to set themselves very high standards.

Goose

 Developing Goose people are self-sacrificing in their determination to achieve their ambitions, and possess and degree of endurance that enables them to accept hardship willingly to attain their goal.

 Developed Goose has the capacity to lead others, and is usually well-organized, clear-sighted, and very determined.

 Extroverted Goose is pragmatic and has an ability to accept seemingly adverse situations and to turn them into advantages for themselves and others with whom they are associated.

 Introverted Goose people tend to be pessimistic and rather severe in their approach. They are likely to be narrow-minded in their outlook and difficult to live with.

Otters

Developing Otters, though gregarious and sociable, are not so readily carried away by their enthusiasms. They have a greater capacity for understanding.

Developed Otters strive after humanitarian ideals and social justice. They have a strong sense of fairness.

Extroverted Otters have deep-rooted convictions and a reforming zeal that is directed to the service of others. They have a selfless devotion to what they believe in.

Introverted Otters are likely to be resentful of any form of restriction or limitation, and rebellious of authority of any kind. They have a strong concept of freedom, but are likely to be very self-centred.

Wolves

Developing Wolves are idealistic and philanthropic with strong spiritual aspirations.

Developed Wolves are gentle, kindly, and compassionate. They have a capacity to demonstrate love by their very actions and lifestyle. They are creative and innovative.

Extroverted Wolves are emotionally sensitive and impressionable. They are self-sacrificing and likely to absorb the suffering of others into themselves, and this makes them vulnerable.

Introverted Wolves have a tendency to want to retreat from the situation they are in after a time and in this way rebuild their strength. They have a strong ability to understand others but are themselves often not understood.

Determining which phase you are in and observing which stage of unfoldment others are at, provides you with a clearer insight into the human condition and a deeper understanding of personality and behaviour.

The Personality Modes

ACCORDING TO THE ELEMENTAL TECHNOLOGY OF THE ANCIENTS, yang, the masculine principle which is evident throughout all Nature, operates through Fire and Air, as the activator and mover of energy, while yin, the feminine principle, works through elemental Water and Earth, as the shaper and solidifier of energy.

The gender of the birth totem – that is, whether it is principally yin or yang – is an indication of the way energies are being expressed through the personality.

Bear in mind that 'masculine' yang is in no way superior to 'feminine' yin, or vice versa. Yang does not dominate yin, nor does yin control yang. Both have equality of being. Creation cannot exist without one or the other. They are opposites but they are not 'opposed' to one another in the sense of being in conflict. They balance one another. Each complements and completes the other. It is through their fusion that new life comes into existence.

Gender alternates through the birth 'months' in order that balance and harmony may be maintained and expressed. The *intention* of each individual expression through the twelve categories of personality can, perhaps, be summarized in a word, which I shall call the keyword of the birth totem in order to emphasize the intention of the yin or yang expression. (See table overleaf.)

According to ancient elemental technology, the yang and yin principles operate through the elemental clans to provide another indication of how the Earth influences function through the human personality. These Earth influences act in a way similar to the tides of the Moon; it is not that they *are* the tides of the Moon, but rather that the study of the operation of the tides of the Moon enables us to comprehend more easily the action and nature of the Earth influences in their operation.

If we regard the four phases of the Moon as modes, or methods

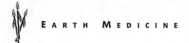
of working, and keep in mind what we have already learned from the four 'faces' of the Moon, we should readily comprehend this deeper aspect of how the qualities and characteristics of the energies 'work'.

	Keyword (Intention)	Gender (Expression)
Falcon	Action	Yang
Beaver	Possession	Yin
Deer	Versatility	Yang
Woodpecker	Devotion	Yin
Salmon	Rulership	Yang
Brown Bear	Practicality	Yin
Crow	Justice	Yang
Snake	Introspection	Yin
Owl	Objectivity	Yang
Goose	Trust	Yin
Otter	Imagination	Yang
Wolf	Understanding	Yin

Let us, then, consider the Moon in its four modes:

THE WAXING MODE

 The Waxing Moon is where the energies are fast-flowing. This mode is connected with making things *work*, with effort and enterprise. Its stress is on facing facts and with overcoming obstacles and difficulties through endeavour.

THE FULL MOON MODE

  The Full Moon mode has to do with culmination, with the climaxing of ideas and efforts, of bringing things to fruition.

THE WANING MODE

 The Waning Moon mode is an *outgoing* of energies. It is a letting go of what is no longer required. It is connected with the service of others and with the resolution of situations.

THE DARK MOON MODE

The Dark Moon mode is the withdrawal of energy. It is the mode of contemplation of what has been performed and consideration of potentialities. It is connected with exploring possibilities.

We can now look at the elemental clans and the birth totems (personality categories) that comprise them, and through our understanding of the Elements of the yang and yin concept, arrive at the principal function of each clan grouping. We can then go on to see the part each personality category has to play within that grouping. (See table on page 266).

Within this structure, functions will be expressed in one of four modes similar to the four 'faces' or phases of the Moon. The Waxing Moon (the Maiden) is indicative of the ones within a clan who are the initiators and creators, the Full Moon (the Mother) is indicative of the ones who are the consolidators and secure and complete things, the Waning Moon (the Grandmother) is indicative of the ones who are the changers and who modify and make perfect. The Dark Moon (Old Woman) is indicative of people of each clan who reflect and express the energies negatively, and whom we might call the Negators. Individuals will express their many qualities in all of the above ways at the same time. No one, for instance, is all negative.

This is a cyclic or circular pattern. It can be approached at the Dark Moon aspect first indicating a negative clearing away to prepare for the work of practical construction and of modification with the purpose of making perfect.

Let me emphasize once again that the Moon is not itself the source of these characteristics, only an indicator of the ebb and flow of their energies. Similarly, the twelve birth totems and personality groupings and Earth influences, together with their modes and phases, are linked to solar dates, but this is not to imply that the Sun is their source. The Sun is a powerful influence on them and they relate to it as the main energy source although the solar energy is modified and conditioned by the Earth and the totems.

The relationship between the Moon's phases, the elemental clans and the birth totems is shown in the table overleaf.

But just as each section is affected by the tides of the Moon however they occur in it, and Nature works with these tides, so we too, as personalities, can learn to work with the tides that are 'conditioning' us.

The duration of these tides in Nature varies, however. The Dark of the

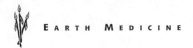

PHASE ➡	Maiden Waxing Moon CREATORS	Mother Full Moon CONSOLIDATORS	Grandmother Waning Moon CHANGERS	Old Woman Dark Moon NEGATORS
BUTTERFLY CLAN The enthusiastic thinkers AIR	Crow thinks up ideas	Otter carries ideas through	Deer jumps from one idea to another and tries to work on many ideas	Negative Butterfly does not discuss. Argues with every thing. Does not communicate ideas
HAWK CLAN The inspiring doers FIRE	Falcon starts things off	Salmon does it	Owl jumps from one thing to another	Negative Hawk does nothing and prevents others from doing anything
FROG CLAN The intuitive feelers WATER	Woodpecker gets involved emotionally	Snake gets involved mentally	Wolf moves from one involvment to another	Negative Frog does not get involved. Not caring
TURTLE CLAN The practical constructors EARTH	Goose prepares the ground and the foundations for new projects. Builds	Beaver secures the framework. Completes	Brown Bear moves around adding a piece here and there. Modifies	Negative Turtle destroys or demolishes. Clears away the old

Moon is only four days, the Waxing Moon covers a period of eleven days, the Full Moon is for only three days, and the Waning Moon lasts eleven days.

You can tune yourself in to the actual Moon phases and discover how they are affecting you personally by observing what is happening both around you and within you during each phase.

Keep a record. Most page-a-day diaries give the dates of the New Moon and Full Moon for the year ahead, and some give the dates, too, of each phase of the Moon. Such a diary can be used as a spiritual notebook. But even an exercise book will do for recording situations which arise at the time of the New Moon and Full Moon in particular, and your reactions to them.

Note also the things you want to bring into your life and the day the desire came into your mind. Record eventually what actually happened about those desires. I don't mean the subjects of fantasizing and day-dreaming, like becoming a millionaire overnight through luck on the pools or gambling, or gaining instant recognition or fame, or being drooled over by a pop-star or TV idol. I mean those desires that are within the range of practical possibility and which you yourself can make determined efforts to bring about.

What you are recording is the outset of a willed desire and of its ultimate outcome, and over a period of time discovering that those desires that are actually satisfied are the ones that 'catch the tide' of the Moon's cycles, and the ones that are frustrated are those whose timing goes against the flow of energies.

You can work consciously with these tides. Again, keep a record. Make a note of new plans begun, and when they come to manifestation. Note down, also, any attempt to get rid of unwanted situations and circumstances.

Three nights from the time of the *New Moon* is the time for generating new ideas and for beginning new projects.

From the fourth night and throughout the *Waxing Moon* to the night before the Full Moon is the period when the Moon's energies influence the emotions and the tides of growth, so this is the time to put effort and feeling into the projects you are working on and the plans you want to bring about.

Though there is plenty of light at the time of the *Full Moon*, the lunar power has reached full blossom and is about to fade. So this is the time for completing what was begun at the New Moon.

Elemental Clan	Element	Gender		
BUTTERFLY Deer Crows Otters	Air	Yang	**Function:** The *distributors* of energy. **Tendency:** Mobility and spontaneity.	
HAWK Falcons Salmon Owls	Fire	Yang	**Function:** The *converters* of energy. **Tendency:** to want things now. Immediacy.	
FROG Woodpeckers Snakes Wolves	Water	Yin	**Function:** The *mergers* of energy. **Tendency:** the need to be involved and to experience.	
TURTLE Beavers Brown Bears Geese	Earth	Yin	**Function:** The *organizers* of energy. **Tendency:** to make things work.	

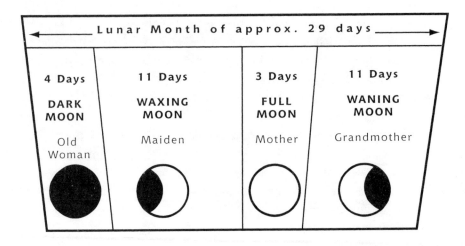

Figure 43.

The period of the *Waning Moon* is the time for making changes and for disposing of things, for bringing things to an end, and for banishing troubles and unwanted conditions.

The last four nights of the Old Moon is when the dark side of the Moon is facing the Earth. This is a good time for meditation and for seeking wisdom and guidance, and for rest.

By synchronizing with the lunar cycles you put yourself more in tune with cosmic energies also, and thereby gain more control of your life and the attainment of greater success and fulfilment.

Totems – the Symbolic Sensors

T HERE IS A SUBLIMINAL NETWORK BETWEEN ALL FORMS OF LIFE which enables an interchange of information to take place between them. Totems act as symbolic sensors in tapping into this network. The Amerindian found that totems served as connectors between different levels of awareness whether human, animal, vegetable or mineral.

In Nature there are three kingdoms 'below' humanity – Animal, Plant and Mineral – and all four are interconnected and interdependent. The plant kingdom is nourished by trace elements from the mineral kingdom and absorbs these minerals into itself and by so doing provides a means for 'inert' minerals to 'evolve' and move through a 'higher' life form and expression. Similarly, the plant kingdom provides sustenance for the animal kingdom and furthers its own development.

The fourth kingdom – the human – is dependent on minerals, plants and animals for its survival. Indeed, the human being comprises elements from all three 'lower' kingdoms, just as the animal comprises plants and minerals, and the plant minerals. Each higher order characterizes the items it consumes so they become more complex elements of itself.

In Nature, it can be observed that everything exists for something else. Everything, in fact, gives of itself and everything receives to itself. The Sun gives its light and heat so that the Earth may have life. The Earth gives of itself to the plants and trees and vegetation, which give themselves to animals and birds and creatures that crawl and swim. And they give themselves to humanity. And all die and give themselves back to the Earth out of which they sprang and were formed, and the cycle of Nature goes on. The circle is completed.

The kingdoms are *states of existence*. So when we use a totem we have a link with another state of existence which can help to condition our own. These states of existence are not entirely external to ourselves as they may appear. They are an integral *part* of ourselves, for though we are humans we contain within the human energy system elements of the mineral, plant and animal kingdoms. Each plays an essential and vital role in the dynamics of our own individual solar system – the little universe that revolves around the 'Sun' that is our individuated self. When we enlist help from these 'kingdoms' in furthering our progress we are extending our understanding and comprehension of the way Nature works, and helping to raise these other forms of consciousness towards a 'higher' nature. We become participators and partners in joint spiritual 'evolution' on our Earth Walk – our terrestrial journey.

A totem is a means of alignment with other levels of being. It is a means of linking one's own organism with energy sources and formative forces that are beyond external manifestation and the range of appearances.

Animal Totems

An animal totem mirrors aspects of our *own* nature, and partly for this reason: the animal kingdom comprises the husbanders of the Earth and forms the link between the plant kingdom and the mineral kingdom. The three together provide a harmonious Earth environment for they balance the atmosphere and the fertility of the planet and provide the ideal conditions to support human life. The extermination of whole species of animals and the exploitation of others has gravely weakened the link, and the delicate balance of Nature is being upset. This is not only harming the Earth but threatening the survival also of the entire human race.

Regretfully, much of humanity regards the animal kingdom as unfeeling matter that can be used for whatever purpose it sees fit. Animals reared for food by factory farming methods or for experimentation to further scientific or medical 'research' can be subjected to horrendous suffering for the use of humanity. Through greed, humanity in general chooses to remain ignorant.

Animals – all animals, whether they run, crawl, swim or fly – have a conscious awareness like you and me. They suffer pain like you and me. They have a love for their young, like you and me. They are feeling, intelligent, living creatures whose guidance system is predominantly instinctive, and who have much to teach us if we will only watch, respect, listen and learn.

Look around for some tangible representations of the animals that are your totems. A totem does not have to be claw, tooth, fur or feather, though fishing tackle shops which sell items for fly-fishing are one source of possible supply for feathers or fur of some animals. You may need to stretch your imagination, but a representation does not have to come directly from the creature itself. The representation serves merely as a tangible link with the qualities and energies the totem represents and a vital means of getting through to the subconscious mind. It serves, also, as a valuable aid to meditation, and for developing the intuitive senses. Intuition is information that comes from *within* and a totem token held in the hand or used as a point of focus whilst meditating can advance such progress.

Browse around gift shops, general stores, shops that sell dress accessories, craft shops, and market stalls. My Eagle is an attractive pendant. My Mouse is a charming porcelain miniature that really captures the character of the little creature. Some may be a little more difficult to acquire unless you live in the United States or Canada. I have clippings from the fur of a grizzly which were given to me, but a taxidermist might help in your search. I obtained the shed skin of a snake from a local zoo. A totem can be represented by a small picture, a visual representation on a ring, or thimble, or any small item of artwork or crafting.

This search is part of the process of tuning your inner senses. Once that process has begun you may be surprised by how just the right thing comes to your attention unexpectedly and how often 'coincidence' seems to be playing a part in your life. It is the working of the subconscious links.

Plant Totems

Study the nature of the plant or tree that is your totem of the plant kingdom. Find out the surroundings it prefers, the kind of soil in which it thrives, the conditions it likes and dislikes, how it responds to change, whether it transplants safely from one place to another, the kind of plants it mixes well with, the phase of the Moon that is best for its planting, and so on. In so doing you will discover facets of your own nature.

Try to discern the auras of plants and trees. Trees and plants each have their own aura. If you look at a plant or tree silhouetted against the sky you may discern a fuzzy glow around it. Just before dusk you might see little swirls of energy around the leaves as they grasp the last rays of the sunlight. Remember, animals express themselves and they move about as we do. Plants and trees express themselves in one place and do not move, hence they can tell us a lot about the place in which they grow.

If your plant totem is easily available, it is best to go out into the countryside and obtain a cutting, or a twig if the totem is a shrub. If this is difficult, try a nursery or a herbal store. Otherwise, a small picture or other representation of the plant will suffice. My thistle totem is the flower-head embedded into a clear plastic dome which I discovered in a craft shop among similar items being sold as small paperweights. Remember, though, if cutting a plant or shrub to tell the plant the purpose for which you need it. It will indicate telepathically which piece may be taken. Place your finger where you will cut and give the plant or shrub time to withdraw its life-force. Afterwards, spit on the fingers and wipe over the bare cut surface as a thankyou and to prevent infection in the plant as spit contains an antiseptic.

Mineral Totems

The mineral kingdom not only provides the substance for the body, which is the physical expression of ourselves, but the food we eat contains elements from the mineral kingdom that provide us with vital and essential needs that enable us to function on the Earth.

Stones and rocks are part of this Earth, and were here long before plants, animals and humans appeared. They have experienced the evolution of the planet itself, and the vast geological and atmospheric changes as Age has succeeded Age. They were around through the rise and fall of civilizations and great empires. They have absorbed much good and bad.

Humanity has always regarded some stones as 'precious'. Nowadays the most 'precious' stones are those which have a scarcity value and, therefore, a greater monetary worth.

But stones were valued by the Amerindian and by ancient peoples not out of material considerations, but because of the energies which were channelled through them. In some way, each stone was a receiver and transmitter of energy that could be used in many ways – for healing, for protection, for channelling thought vibrations, for tuning in to psychic patterns, for meditation, and many more.

Just as we each have something in common with our blood relations, however near or distant they may be, because something in our genes, perhaps, binds us together as 'family' and enables us to be supportive and share a sense of 'belonging', so we have an affinity with a gemstone.

A gemstone, too, is a 'relative', but one that exists in a 'lower' – or, rather, denser – realm of existence, though it is one that, to an extent, interpenetrates our own. There is a similarity that extends beyond the material –

a similarity of *qualities*.

A gemstone can help the human being to enhance and develop the qualities they share. The human being, in enlisting the help of a gemstone, enables it, too, to elevate its own evolutionary development because it is given the opportunity to participate in the awareness of a being with a 'higher' level of consciousness.

A crystal, for instance, is more highly evolved in its path of evolution than any human is in his.

The selection of stones as totems in this book are those revealed to me by Silver Bear and represent twelve potential characteristics of humanity. They should not be compared with the birthstones of Sun astrology or so-called 'lucky' stones. Each has practical value in developing the virtues assigned to them. They operate in ways similar to the chakras of the energy body – as connectors or transformers between different levels – in bringing into manifestation the characteristics they symbolize.

There is thus a great difference between a gemstone used as a mineral totem and a 'lucky' birthstone. A birthstone is generally regarded as an inanimate object which through an association with certain planetary vibrations is able to draw 'magnetically' fortunate influences to the one who wears it.

The gemstone totem, on the other hand, was regarded by the American Indians as a manifestation of the Great Everything and an organism with 'aliveness', though very different from our own. The stone generates subtle energies which are related to human qualities and virtues. These qualities, in either their positive or negative aspect, are an integral part of humans born at a particular period in the Earth's yearly cycle. Each personality category exhibits something of the related gemstone characteristics or a need for the qualities it emphasizes.

Gemstones given in this book can be obtained fairly easily from dealers in semi-precious stones, from some department stores, and specialist shops. Wherever possible let intuition be your guide in your choice of stone. I am told that ideally it is not a matter of us choosing a stone, but of the stone choosing its humans partner.

If you are presented with a tray of similar stones, or see several exhibited or on display, don't be persuaded by what a salesperson or someone else may say, nor by the physical appearance alone of a particular stone. Seek inner guidance in making your choice and you will understand what I mean. Bear in mind that it is the inner harmony of the stone you are seeking to contact and to work with.

Your totem stone is going to be of particular importance to you because it is on your own 'wavelength' and shares certain of your attributes or is able to connect you with what you lack or require. It is going to be your connection with the mineral kingdom, so the selection is important. Ask to hold a stone that appeals to you. Hold it in your left hand (which is your *receiving* hand) and scan over it with your other hand (your giving hand). You may be able to feel its power. Ask yourself mentally, 'Is this the stone that is right for me?' Your True Self knows. So let your True Self be your guide.

Any stone you acquire will have passed through many hands and been in contact with many different environments, so it is necessary to cleanse it of any negative vibrations. This is done simply by putting it into a glass containing a solution of clean water and a pinch of salt with, perhaps, a teaspoonful of cider vinegar for a while. Then hold it under running water from a tap or in a stream. Afterwards leave it for a day or two on a shelf where it can bathe in the sunlight or moonlight.

Next, the stone has to be 'awakened' or attuned to you. This, again, is simple. Just hold it in the palm of one hand and think and feel love into it. If it helps, think of love as a ball of energy around it. Ask the 'spirit' within the stone to work with you. You may feel a response from the stone if you cup your other hand over it gently and close your eyes. It may be a gentle warmth, a slight tingling sensation, or even a slight pulsation.

This same procedure can be adopted for any further stones you acquire, and especially with crystals. Then, respect and treasure them: don't just hide them away. Expose them to the sunlight or moonlight. Let them add their lustre to the aura of your home. If you want to carry one around with you, put it in a soft little pouch or bag.

The Amerindian shaman regarded stones as living beings that aided him in his multidimensional activities and extended the range of his extrasensory abilities.

Once you have chosen and 'activated' your stone in the way I have described and had it with you for a time you will discover for yourself what a valuable aid you have.

This, of course, is true of all your totems which serve as 'helpers' in bringing you into harmony with the Earth rather than in conflict with it, and by so doing restoring the harmony your own energy-system craves.

How to Obtain Your Own 'Readings'

ONE OF THE BIG ATTRACTIONS OF EARTH MEDICINE IS THAT IT does not require the setting up of natal charts or any complex astrological calculations. With Earth Medicine you work with Nature, not an ephemeris.

Earth Medicine is a system that puts its user into contact with Nature and with the Earth's natural cycles. As we have seen, it occasions a study of the phases of the Moon as indicators of how the Earth influences are flowing. It can become a highly personalized system because it exercises and develops the user's own intuitive senses and restores the vital lost contact with the Inner Self and with Earth. It most importantly provides an understanding of why all is as it is, and it engenders a love and respect for Mother Earth as our guardian and teacher.

So let us get down to some practical work and build up some 'Readings' in stages.

Say we want to seek guidance for a particular day. The first step is to check the date with the Earth Web to determine the time section in which it falls and its position within that section – that is, whether it comes at or near its beginning or end or its middle.

For instance, say the date we have in mind is 24 March. By referring to the Earth Web we find that 24 March comes in the time-section 21 March – 19 April, which is Awakening Time. The totem for that period is Falcon.

I have explained elsewhere that the Time conditions to an extent the quality of the days its period embraces, and that the name allocated to each time-period describes a feature of its essence. The Awakening Time is when spring is in the air, and Nature is bursting forth into new life. So put yourself in harmony with Nature's own cycle by getting a 'feel' of that particular time-cycle and what it means to you.

Since 24 March comes near the beginning to the Awakening Time cycle it might suggest a day for new beginnings and for putting one's heart into some new endeavour towards a brighter future ahead. Let me stress that this is my own reaction in attempting to capture the 'feel' of the day in relation to its position in time. You must arrive at your own interpretation. I am deliberately avoiding suggesting any hard and fast rules. The important thing is to keep an open mind and to be relaxed. Allow yourself to 'connect' with Nature and with Mother Earth. Don't 'try'. You don't have to make an effort. Relax, and wait expectantly for a response. Thoughts and words appropriate to the day will come to you. Write them down immediately. They are the 'stuff' with which to work. Try not to 'read' them as you write. Just let the pen flow until you stop – then put the pen down and read.

Having thus captured the 'mood' of the day, the next step is to determine the flow of Earth influences and how they are likely to affect that condition. Since it is the phases of the Moon that gives an indication of the way the Earth influences are flowing, we need to ascertain which of the four phases applies to the day being examined.

Most daily newspapers record the phase of the Moon in their weather forecast. Monthly horoscope magazines provide useful information on what the Moon is doing for the month ahead. But if you want to look further ahead you will need a good diary which gives at least the New Moon and Full Moon dates for the entire year – or, better still, an Almanac or Moon Calendar. Such items are available from most 'New Age' bookshops.

What we need to know is whether the day being examined comes under the mode of the Dark Moon, the Waxing Moon, the Full Moon, or the Waning Moon. When we have that information we can take our understanding a stage further.

For the sake of example, let us suppose that 24 March falls during the four days of the Dark Moon. Remember, the days of the Dark Moon are easy to find because they cover the four days immediately preceding the New Moon. So with 24 March falling within the four-day span of the Dark Moon, what might that suggest? A day for introspection and rest from outgoing activity, perhaps? A day best suited to nurturing seeds of ideas or new plans. A day for considering potentials rather than getting too involved in aggressive activity.

Remember, it is not the Moon alone that is affecting such things. The Moon is giving an indication of how the Earth influences are operating, and in this example those Earth influences are in a state of pause, just like our breathing at that point when air has been expelled from the lungs but we have not yet begun to inhale again. It might also be described as a 'holding' of that which might come forth into new activity.

Now if we consider what we have already written about the 'mood' of the time on 24 March and let our mind relax into considering how those tendencies might operate under a Dark Moon we may find ourselves writing something like this:

> 24 March would appear to be a day in which to consider carefully hopes for the immediate future and for thinking of practical ways in which they might be implemented. If you do that, then you should be able to push ahead in a few days with confidence, knowing that the future will be bright.

Now we must consider the third factor in the build-up of a 'Reading' – the totem of the time section in which the chosen date appears. For 24 March it is Falcon, in the Northern hemisphere.

Bear in mind that the totem embraces the characteristics of the total Earth influence for that time as reflected in the personality. So refer back to the relevant section in Part Two which considers the qualities of the birth and animal totem. This is located in subsection 7.

One of the characteristics of Falcon is that it is a far-sighted bird that sees things from afar. That attribute throws further light on our 'Reading' for 24 March which might now be amended:

> 24 March is a day for planning ahead to implement your hopes for the immediate future. Consider carefully practical ways to accomplish your plans, then you can push ahead with confidence in a few days knowing that the future will be bright.

Let us take a second example, for those born in the Northern hemisphere, say 18 July. This date comes in the period 21 June – 21 July in the Long Days Time. Its totem is Woodpecker.

In checking the date with the Earth Web we find it comes near the end of the Long Days Time. This is the period of midsummer when the days are usually hot and the Sun is at its strongest, when dawn comes early and dusk comes late so the days appear to be 'stretched out'.

Since 18 July comes near the transition from one time section to the next, there is a pull towards the time just ahead which, in this case, is the Ripening Time when Nature is coming to its fruition. Again, try to catch the 'mood' of this period of time. It may suggest that 18 July is a day for you to slow down a bit and enjoy what you're doing, bearing in mind that efforts of the past that have taken root and have been developing will shortly bear fruit. In other words, this isn't a day for getting all tensed up!

Again, this is an indication, not a dogmatic statement. Your intuitive sense may suggest a rather different emphasis and one that is intended for *you*. The aim is not to attain an identical 'Reading' with someone else, but to get yourself in tune with Nature and the cycle of time in question so that your own intuitive senses come into play to provide clues to the way the Earth influences are meaningful to you.

The knowledge you need comes from within you, not from some outside source.

Now let us apply the Moon mode principle to 18 July. This time for the purpose of example let us suppose that 18 July falls as the Moon is at its next stage and is New and beginning to wax.

The 'mood' of the time for 18 July indicated that past efforts would bear fruit if one slowed down a bit and took advantage of the 'stretched out' day. Since a Waxing Moon is when the tides of Earth influences are flowing toward fulfilment, we might expand on what was previously written with something like this:

> 18 July is a day to flow with the tide and to revel in the experience. The efforts of the past will soon find fulfilment if you let go and just 'let it happen'.

Now we check with the totem for that period. What strikes us about the Woodpecker? Woodpeckers perform out of sheer enjoyment but need comfort and security. So, bearing this characteristic in mind, our 'Reading' for 18 July might now be something like this:

> 18 July is a day to take comfort from the efforts of the past which will soon be finding fulfilment if you will just 'let them happen' and don't get in the way. So, enjoy the moment. Don't live in the past, or anticipate the future. Enjoy the moment. Flow with today's tide and revel in the experience.

As our next example let us take at random 28 October which we find comes in the period 23 October – 22 November. Its totem is Snake. The date comes a quarter of the way through the Frost Time. What does the Frost Time suggest? Crisp, cold, snappy mornings that have a bite in the air. A time when only hardy plants survive Jack Frost's penetrating chill. In its negative action, Frost destroys, but it quickly retreats and vanishes when exposed to warmth. In its positive action, Frost breaks down the soil and helps transform and prepare it for the seed of the new life that is to come.

So, 28 October suggests to me a day to be crisp and brief and direct in my dealings – otherwise my tasks may not be brought to a completion. A day, perhaps, on which to break things down to their basic components in preparing the ground for long-term projects.

Let us assume that 28 October falls within the next Moon mode – that is, during the three days of the Full Moon when the Earth influences reach their peak. Putting these factors together we might now come up with something like this:

> 28 October is a day when past endeavours reach their peak. The lessons learned from them should be looked at critically and broken down to form the substance for completing long-term projects.

Now we consult the totem for the Frost Time. Snake is a creature that sheds its skin frequently and is associated with transformation. This quality helps to further our 'Reading' for 28 October. Something like this, perhaps:

> 28 October is a day when past endeavours have reached their peak. The lessons learned from them should be looked at critically and quickly broken down to form the substance for completing long-term projects which will transform your life.

As a further example we will take 29 December, which falls within the time-section 22 December – 19 January and is called the Renewal Time. Its totem is Goose.

This date comes mid-way through the Renewal Time, which is a period for rest and renewal and refreshment. It is a time for making resolutions, and since 29 December comes at the heart of this period the day should reflect very much the spirit of its time.

I would gather from this that 29 December is a day on which to relax and to put aside those things that have served their purpose in the past but are no longer truly relevant. It suggests to me renewal – making 'new' again – so perhaps it is a good day to consider those elements of the past months which have been of proven value and which, therefore, should form the basis of resolutions that could help determine the future.

Now to check with what the Moon is doing on that day. Let us suppose that 29 December falls during the period when the Moon is waning. Remember, a waning Moon indicates that the tides of Earth influences are moving away from us and is thus a period suited not only for getting rid of things we don't want but of a giving of things that we value. This seems to strengthen what we had sensed from the 'mood' of the time. So we might write something like this:

> 29 December is a day to begin making a complete break with those things in the past that have now served their purpose. It is a day for making new resolutions from the lessons the past has taught you, particularly those faults you want to give up.

Now we check with the totem animal – Goose. Goose is associated with purity of intent and with sheer determination. This helps our further understanding, so our 'Reading' might now become:

> 29 December is a day to begin making a complete break with those things of my past that have now served their purpose and are no longer valid. It is a day for making new resolutions from the lessons the past has taught me, and for ensuring the purity of their intention so that I can push them through with determination to attain my aim. With purity of heart and firm intent, I give up my faults that I now recognize.

One further set of examples should help you to obtain a thorough grasp of the principles involved. Let us take one more date – say 17 March – and see what different interpretations are arrived at when we apply the characteristics of each of the Moon modes to the 'mood' of the time.

In checking the Earth Web we find that 17 March comes near the end of the Blustery Winds Time and shortly before Awakening Time. The Blustery Winds Time, as its name suggests, is that period in the yearly cycle when we may have to literally 'hold on to our hats' as we struggle against the strong, swirling gusts of wind that seem intent on wanting to snatch them from us.

The 'feeling' I get is that this is a period when it seems right to expect the unexpected to happen. It is also a time to be on one's guard against having things that are in reach snatched from one's grasp. It is a day when we need, perhaps, to hold things closely to us.

The totem is Wolf, an animal that is at home on the mountains as well as on the plains.

Consider these pointers and how they might operate under each of the four Moon modes. This is what comes to me:

Dark Moon: 17 March is a day to stop struggling and wasting your energies. It is a day for reflection and for taking stock, and for preparing yourself for the calmer days just ahead when you will more easily be able to obtain what you want without having to struggle every inch of the way. Like the Wolf, learn to choose the right time to act. This is not such a day. Practise acceptance.

Waxing Moon: 17 March is a day to stick with it and not allow yourself to be blown off course or diverted. The going may seem rough, but hold on to what you know to be right and keep your head. Things will calm down very soon and all your efforts will prove worthwhile if you will stick with it and don't lose sight of your goal.

Full Moon: 17 March is a day to keep your feet firmly on the ground. The winds of change have been blowing through your life and causing you concern and even discomfort. But you should find that if you concentrate on practicalities rather than fantasizing on things beyond reach, they will help to bring your hopes to fulfilment. Be one with the winds of change.

Waning Moon: Don't hold on selfishly to things that may appear to be important to you. Let others share your good fortune. Unless you are willing to pass on to others some of the benefits you have derived from your experiences, you may even find them suddenly taken from you. This day has the message that there is happiness in giving as well as joy in having. Be a distributor with the winds.

Now have a go at formulating a 'Reading' for yourself. Take today's date. Your daily newspaper should indicate which mode of the Moon is in operation today if you are not already aware of it. Then put your intuitive senses to work. You don't have to 'try hard' or put 'effort' into it. Just relax and let it happen. The words will come to you if you just simply absorb yourself in the spirit of the Time and the relevant Moon mode and totem animal.

Act on whatever evidence you obtain in your 'Reading'. Your confidence in the system will increase when the results of such actions become apparent.

Keep a record. Read today's reading again tomorrow and compare it with the day you actually had. Write up 'Readings' for members of your family and let them participate. You will soon come to realize what a valuable tool you have acquired for practical, everyday living.

The method I have outlined here measures the mood and essence of the

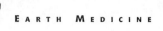

day; it does not predict an individual's possible response to it. Free will is left unhampered. It is like a weather forecast. You are free to determine whether or not to take a raincoat with you when you venture out of doors; the forecast does not prophesy whether or not you will get drenched.

An even finer tuning that can indicate the likely response of the individual to the mood of the day can be obtained by applying characteristics of the Birth Totem to the 'reading' and also of the Influencing Elements. It is best, however, to get experience of the basic method before attempting this, since the skills involved are largely intuitive and take time to develop.

Travelling the Web

YOUR BIRTH TOTEM SHOWS YOUR VIEWING-POINT ON LIFE FROM your starting-place in space and time where your life's journey on Earth began. The collection of associated totems indicates the potentials and qualities you were equipped to work with.

In discovering your totems through Earth Medicine you come to know and understand yourself more and become encouraged to take control of your life. With that knowledge will come a realization that there are qualities you appear to lack, or have neglected or overlooked. That realization is as important to you as the recognition of the assets you do possess as an individual, for what you lack is what you need to attain balance and bring harmony into your life. You need to travel the Circle of the Medicine Web to find that balance and harmony.

Some totems are the equivalent of what psychologists have called 'archetypes'. An archetype is an animated symbol, a pattern or model that indicates how certain forces are operating in one's life and what one's relationship with them is. It is a living energy that contains patterns of behaviour that make up the impersonal part of the psyche, or what Jungian psychologists call the Collective Unconscious which all of us share.

In Western cultures, archetypes are usually presented in human form, each expressing masculine or feminine characteristics. They figure as characters in myths and legends, as gods and goddesses, and as the actors in fairy-tales and folk-stories. Each embraces knowledge and possesses certain qualities and characteristics. These combine to give them their power, or what the Amerindian would described as their 'medicine'.

With animal, plant and mineral totems, gender is not imputed, so the fundamental essence of the quality is presented in a neutral state and before expression as either masculine or feminine, positive or negative. Since animals, plants and rocks existed on Earth before humanity appeared, the Amerindian concluded they were therefore nearer to the origins of Earth life.

Similarly, animal, plant and mineral totems were seen as being closer to the source of a human being's life and, therefore, essential to the understanding of it for they are within us and part of us.

Each of your totems will have something you have, too, and perhaps something you are not making use of, and something you need. Each will have something you have to learn. Each can lead you to a fuller understanding of yourself, because the overriding purpose of a totem is to help you to find your own 'medicine' or power.

The totems, then, are 'teachers'. When you connect with a totem you are establishing not just an affinity with an archetype, but a communication with the symbolism inherent in it. Symbolism, not words, is the language of the subconscious mind. It is the substance of the imagination. It is the sensing device of the intuition. So totems enable you to have access to your deeper self and to come to know that aspect of your being more fully.

By 'travelling' the Medicine Web you are building up your connections with the Earth and coming into balance and harmony with everything around you and within you, for the Medicine Web connects you to the infinity of life within the Great Everything and to the centre of your own being.

We each of us enter life at our respective starting-points on the Web depending on the month or time of our birth. We come equipped with certain attributes and potentials, traits and qualities, strengths and weaknesses, and these are expressed in the totems of Beavers, Deer, Snakes, Otters, Wolves, and so on.

We are born into a particular elemental clan. Our clan has nothing to do with our physical family relationships, but with the element we are most closely related to and have a responsibility for. We share the qualities of that element with other clan relatives, though those qualities will operate and be expressed in different way.

For instance, Falcons, Salmon and Owls share the characteristics of elemental Fire in the Hawk Clan. Beavers, Brown Bears and Geese share the characteristics of elemental Earth in the Turtle Clan. Deer, Crows and Otters share the characteristics of elemental Air in the Butterfly Clan, and Woodpeckers, Snakes and Wolves share the characteristics of elemental Water in the Frog Clan. And as we have seen in Chapters 7 and 8 each is creator or initiator, consolidator or changer of the energies being expressed through that element.

To stay in your starting-place all through your life would mean that you would hardly grow and develop. That is the problem with most people. They grow only in accordance with their physical development – from infant to child, from child to youth, from youth to adult, and from adulthood to old age. That is one reason why so many people feel dissatisfied and frustrated and somehow 'missing out' on the good things of life. Their growth has been stunted. Their life has no purpose. They are gripped in the quicksand of their own limitations, seemingly not getting anywhere for the simple reason that they are not going anywhere. They are bored with their routine existence. Their lives lack movement and excitement. They find escape only through watching television – through the hours of electronic fantasy, the manufactured world of make-believe that becomes their reality. They may look to their horoscopes for signs of getting out of the quagmire they're in, and though they may regard popular astrology as just 'a bit of fun' they make claim to being Aries, Taurus, Virgo, Libra, Scorpio, Pisces, or whatever, and even make their 'sign' an *excuse* for being the way they are.

That is not what was intended for your life. Look around at Nature itself and you will see that life itself is movement and change. In Earth Medicine you learn to come into harmony with that movement and change. In Earth Medicine you are not static. You move about and make changes, and by so doing enlarge and enrich your life. You are not fixed to a sign of the zodiac, but progress round the Web gaining the strengths you need from other positions, experiencing new challenges, and gaining knowledge from its lessons. By choosing to follow the 'medicine' way, you acquire the gifts and powers and attributes from the different places on the Web.

After learning about your own starting-place and getting to know your own totems and your own strengths and weaknesses, you may determine to develop the powers or 'medicines' you already have before moving round to seek others you are lacking.

The Medicine Wheel is based on the solar cycle in which the Sun appears to move in a clockwise direction from east to west, so in Earth Medicine the time-periods succeed one another in a clockwise direction. But moving from one position to the next around the Web is not the only way to travel. You can move to your complementary totem directly opposite your starting-place on the Web with the intention, say, of bringing your attributes into balance. You can with the intention, say, of bringing your attributes into balance. You can move in turn to the two positions that share your elemental clan for the purpose, say, of learning how to express the characteristics you share in a different way or with a different emphasis. Perhaps there is a quality you know you are lacking, and which would make a big improvement in your life were you to develop it. Then look around the Earth Web for it. Examine the summaries at the beginning of each of the twelve segments in Part Two and when you have located the quality you want, check to see which totem is incorporating it, then get to know that totem. You may feel drawn to a particular totem, or find you have an affinity with an animal, plant or gemstone that serves as a totem also. Get to know it. Add it to the ones you already have.

Moving to another place on the Web means learning about its time and its nature and the 'spirit' of its directional power, its elements and its totems. It means observing how people you know who were born in that cycle are expressing its qualities in their own lives.

It is not just a mental exercise. It means endeavouring to apply the principles each position embraces. It means endeavouring to absorb its attributes into your own time.

There is no right or wrong way of travelling the Web. The only right way is the one that seems right to *you*. The important thing is to keep moving, for then you keep developing and growing and as you do so you extend your perceptions and deepen your understanding and come to see life from all points of view. That could take you a lifetime or even several lifetimes. Or you may complete it many times, learning something new with each round, for the Circle will expand as you go. Only you can set the pace.

The advice of my mentors is that one should seek first to balance the elemental powers and the yang and yin polarities which comprise one's inner dynamics, or the basic spiritual alchemy described in Part Two of this work. It is a matter of examining your 'starting' collection of totems which comprise your basic make-up and determine what elements are lacking in order to bring yourself into harmonious balance. If there is a predominance of yang you require yin, and if yin predominates you should seek the balancing factor of yang. What elements are lacking in your section of the Web? If you are, say, Beaver (predominantly yin!) in the east, which has Earth with Fire, then Water and Air are needed. You could look to Wolf, which has Water with Air and is predominantly yang. Brown Bear in the south-south-west has Earth with Water and is predominantly yin, and needs Air and Fire. Deer is Air with Fire and predominantly yang. Or take a birth totem that has only one influencing element, like Otter in the north. Otter is predominant yang and needs Earth, Fire and Water. Fire could be obtained from its complementary Salmon in the South, and Water with Earth from Snake in the west or Earth with Water from Brown Bear in the south-south-west.

Should you be presented with a choice, refer to the summary at the start of each of the birth totems in Part Two and select the one that appears to present the particular qualities you lack and need.

Study the section carefully and concentrate on the quality or qualities you need. Consider how you can apply them in your everyday life. Consider the birth (animal) totem and its characteristics and regard it as 'added' to your starting collection. Use it as a focus of attention in periods of meditation.

A further help can be horoscope books and articles which include summaries of famous people and celebrities and personalities in the public eye. See how they have made use of the qualities and traits of their particular birth totem in achieving what they have and seek to emulate them by applying those same principles in your own life-situations.

The chart on the next page should enable you to identify at a glance the totems to go to.

A next step could be to explore your polarity totem on the opposite side of the Web. So let us briefly examine the polarity pairings.

 # Falcons and Crows

Falcons and Crows are each involved in *beginnings*. Falcon's place on the Earth Web is at the beginning of spring, whereas Crow's is at the beginning of autumn.

Falcon is endowed with potential creativity and the powerful urge for individual activity. But this outpouring of energy into new activity generally lacks the stability of completion. Falcon is a good starter but a poor finisher. So Falcon can learn from Crow, who is good at getting things done, but not so good at getting things started, and vice versa.

Falcon is concerned with self-initiated action and is quick at making individual decisions, but this trait can develop into rashness, impulsiveness and impatience. So Falcon can learn from Crow's sense of balance, of getting things into sensible proportion, and of being tactful and diplomatic. Whereas Falcon is concerned more with the individual self, Crow is involved more with a group, be it family, or an organization or community. Falcon can thus discover how to balance the urge for action with the calm deliberation of Crow and see other's viewpoint just as clearly as his own.

Crows can learn from Falcon by applying something of Falcon's fortitude and capacity for work, and the recognition that compromise is not necessarily the best solution, especially if it entails the abandonment of principle.

Totem	Inherent elements	Polarity emphasized	Elements needed and possible sources
Falcon	Fire	Yang	Earth, Air and Water. Crow (Air with Earth). Brown Bear (Earth with Water).
Beaver	Earth with Fire	Yin	Air and Water. Wolf (Water with Air).
Deer	Air with Fire	Yang	Earth and Water. Brown Bear (Earth with Water) or Snake (Water with Earth).
Woodpecker	Water	Yin	Earth, Fire and Air. Owl (Fire with Earth). Wolf (Water with Air). Goose (Earth with Air).
Salmon	Fire with Water	Yang	Earth and Air. Goose (Earth with Air) or Crow (Air with Earth).
Brown Bear	Earth with Water	Yin	Air and Fire. Deer (Air with Fire).
Crow	Air with Earth	Yang	Fire and Water. Salmon (Fire with Water).
Snake	Water with Earth	Yin	Air and Fire. Deer (Air with Fire).
Owl	Fire with Earth	Yang	Air and Water. Wolf (Water with Air).
Goose	Earth with Air	Yin	Fire and Water. Salmon (Fire with Water).
Otter	Air	Yang	Fire, Earth and Water. Beaver (Earth with Fire) and Snake (Water and Earth).
Wolf	Water with Air	Yin	Fire and Earth. Beaver (Earth with Fire) or Owl (Fire with Earth).

Beavers and Snakes

Beavers are affected by the Growing Time of Spring when Nature comes into full bloom, and Snakes by the period in the yearly cycle when the trees have shed their leaves and Nature looks barren – the Frost Time.

Beavers are endowed with an urge to preserve and conserve. They are security-conscious, and loyalty, devotion and duty are important principles to them. Beavers crave material security and a stable environment in which to accumulate possessions all around them, though this tendency can degenerate into possessiveness and greed. Beavers can learn from Snakes who, rather than amassing, eliminate. Snakes push aside the temporal things they no longer need, and make use of their practical skills for the benefit of others. Beavers can make far more use of their potentials if they will learn from Snakes to look at life more deeply.

Snakes are endowed with an intensity of purpose which enables them to concentrate and focus their desires, but they are prone to let their serious-ness develop into fanaticism. Snakes can learn from Beavers' amiability. Snakes, though good at managing others, are not so good at handling their own affairs and can learn much in this direction from Beavers.

Deer and Owls

Deer is born during the Flowering Time that connects spring with summer, and reflects change by constantly moving from one interest to another. Deer, who is endowed with a good intellect and a desire to communicate ideas, often becomes entangled in a collection of information which serves little practical purpose. Deer can learn much from Owl in training the intellect to bring about desired improvements that will be longer-lasting.

Owl, of the Long Nights Time, has an eye on the long-term future and is frequently being carried away by idealistic notions. Owl needs to relate idealism with practical living, and can learn much from Deer in dealing more immediately with everyday needs.

Woodpecker and Goose

Woodpecker, of the Long Days Time, is concerned with the urge to nourish and with selective sharing. Woodpecker is sensitive, impressionable and highly emotional and acts largely on gut feeling. Woodpecker has much to

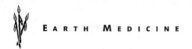

learn from Goose who is more impersonal and objective and whose outlook on life is wider. Goose is of the Renewal Time.

Woodpecker often functions on raw emotion, whereas Goose, who can take on some burdensome responsibilities, runs on an efficiency that arises out of sheer necessity and being a good organizer.

The driving ambition of Goose can lead them to repress their emotions and to appear cold and aloof to others. Goose needs the balance of Woodpecker's more personal and subjective approach and the capture of Woodpecker's desire for a stable base.

 # Salmon and Otters

Salmon, of the Ripening Time, has strength, determination, and a self-expressive nature. Salmon is concerned with the personal use of authority, whereas Otter's interest is in the way the whole community is governed. Salmon seek to better themselves, whereas Otters seek to improve the world. Otter is of the Cleansing Time.

Salmon can be so wrapped up in their own individuality that they fail to respect the individuality of others, and act as if their own way is the only way. Salmon can find balance by learning from Otter's more detached mental outlook. And Otters can help Salmon to find wider scope for their creative energies by recognizing that the individual can never find true fulfilment in isolation.

Otters tend to theorize and fantasize, and their activity is more mental than physical. They need to acquire the sustaining strength of Salmon, and the energy and drive to put their ideas into action.

Otters tend to be more concerned with a group or with things as a whole, rather than the individual, and overlook the fact that any group is but a collection of individuals. They need to learn that an improvement in society can come about only through improved individuals. They can learn from Salmon to develop and balance their own individuality.

 # Brown Bears and Wolves

Brown Bears and Wolves feel impelled to serve, but whereas Bears find their identity through serving others, Wolves tend to lose theirs through the service of others. Brown Bears are of the Harvesting Time.

Bears are practical and like to break things down into manageable components and in this way can cope with quite complex issues. Bear looks at life through a microscope.

Wolves are exceptionally creative because they are endowed with an ability to tap into the imagination more readily than most people. Freedom of movement is essential for their well-being, and they feel a need to break out from the confinement of limitations which restrict this creativity. Wolves are of the Blustery Winds Time.

Wolves see things in their entirety and recognize not so much differences as similarities. They have a wide vision and a deep understanding. Wolf looks at life as if through a telescope.

Bears can gain a wider vision by learning from Wolves to see things as a whole. They need also to acquire something of the compassion and understanding of Wolves to save them from becoming over-critical of others.

Wolves can learn from Bears the importance of detail, and that practicality is important in all creative work. Bears can help Wolves to determine how and when and where to apply their creativity in order to bring about the practical results they desire.

'Centring' Yourself

Before moving to another position on the Web it is important to 'centre' yourself. 'Centring' means going to the centre of the Web.

To be 'centred' means to be aware of the separateness and individualization of the self from the rest of the universe. It means recognition that you are a unique individual. You are you and none other. You will never be duplicated.

But to be 'centred' also means recognizing the limitations of your own human perception and the need to transcend it. That means identifying with something larger than yourself by aligning yourself with the energy-flow of the universe.

'Centring' means balancing ingoing and outgoing forces. It is a form of meditation. It requires the recognition that you are at the centre of your own universe, and that you can also be at one with the infinite power of the universe. Though separate, you are absorbed within it. It is the recognition that a drop of sea water is the same as the ocean that contains it. So it works with you and through you.

When these forces are balanced, a resultant condition comes into being. The Amerindian and the Masters of the Ancient Wisdom called this condition 'illumination'. Illumination is a sudden awareness that strikes like a flash of lightning in the darkness. It is instant realization. It is a sudden flash of insight into something which one had not seen before. It is a flash of light that makes something that was hidden suddenly clear. What then becomes clear to you is a knowledge that is yours. It is knowledge that is personal to you. It becomes your knowledge and your truth, not someone else's that you have 'borrowed' or that has been inflicted on you. That is the kind of knowledge that comes to you through Earth Medicine.

In Earth Medicine, we are no longer cut off from Nature and the elemental forces of the universe, but connected to them, and we find that all things are connected to us. So we are no longer isolated, imprisoned within our own tight little man-made compartments, but free to journey round the Web, discovering not only its magikal wonders but the wonder of our own self as we go. Life has a purpose.

Meditation is means of 'finding the Centre', of discovering your own centre, and by so doing benefiting physically, mentally, emotionally and spiritually.

For meditation to be effective on all four levels of one's being, it is necessary to create four essential conditions. You need to:

- Create the Time.

- Create the Space.

- Create the Power.

- Create the Vision.

Let us examine these four conditions.

1. Create the Time

You have to exert the will to set aside a period in the day to meditate. It can be early in the morning before you set off for work, or begin the routine chores of the day. Even if it means *making* time by getting up half an hour earlier, do it. Early morning is a good time for meditation.

It can be during the day when you can conveniently 'switch off' from your normal work and take time out for a period of secluded relaxation. Or you can choose the evening, when the cares and worries of the day are behind you, and the pressure is off and you are winding down.

2. Create the Space

To meditate effectively you need to find your own space – your own place in the universe which is entirely yours and where you can be free from distraction and interruption. Once established, this space will be uniquely yours. It will be there for you to go to at any time, wherever you are, but first it has to be established on the physical plane.

So, prepare a place in your home. In a spare room perhaps, in a corner of a bedroom, in an attic or basement room – anywhere that no one else is going to be using at that time and where you can be free from disturbance and interruption. The area need only be small, but where you can sit comfortably and have a flat surface in front of you, like a table, a bureau or cupboard top, or perhaps just an empty shelf.

You can make the space your own by burning an incense stick or cone to neutralise the atmosphere for your meditation period and set it apart from mundane activity. You can use a candle as a power switch, so that when the candle is lit at the beginning of your meditation session it indicates to the subconscious mind that the space is switched 'on' for meditation, and when there is no candle light the space is switched 'off' and assigned to any mundane activity. Neither incense nor a candle is necessary, but they can be helpful in setting the right atmosphere.

3. Create the Power

As a preliminary to meditation itself, it is necessary to relax the physical body and the mind and to release any tension that might otherwise block the flow of vital energies through the chakras.

It is best to wear something loose-fitting while meditating so that the body is not restricted in any way, and to remove your shoes.

Sit comfortably, back straight, legs slightly apart, and feet firmly in contact with the floor. Rest the palms of your hands on your knees.

Then *relax the body*. Simply let go of all bodily tensions, starting at the feet and working up to the head.

Relax the mind by *letting go* of all mental worries and anxieties, and all the cares and concerns about your work, your home, your family.

Close your eyes and picture a peaceful beauty spot. If you have a peaceful place where you always feel at ease – a deserted beach by the sea on a warm, sunny day perhaps, or a cool glade in a forest, or by a gently flowing stream, or in an open meadow – just call it to mind. Be there in your imagination, now.

Listen for the sounds of Nature all around you – the gentle lapping of waves on the sand, the song of birds in the trees, the soft dance of flowing water. *Smell* the tang of sea air, the musky freshness of trees, the clear fragrance of grass and heather and wild flowers. *Feel* the soft sand under your feet, or the springiness of grass. Let your imagination activate your inner senses in this way and you will be creating for yourself a beautiful, relaxing mind-space where you can go anytime and be secure, safe and tranquil.

Having now relaxed and found tranquillity in your mind-space, the next stage is to extract cosmic energy from the atmosphere around you and to channel it through the chakras.

We all know that it is breathing that keeps us alive. It has been explained to us at some time that physiologically the process of breathing extracts oxygen from the air when it reaches the lungs and it is then absorbed into the bloodstream and it is this that keeps up alive.

But there is another element in the air which modern medical science does not recognize because it cannot be seen or measured. I have referred to it earlier as prana or mana. The Chinese call it *chi* and the Japanese *Ki*. Whatever word is used, it means 'life-force'. It is not physical substance but pure spirit-energy. It permeates all things and supports every atom, keeping everything that is in existence shimmering and vibrating. It is that which makes possible all organic functions, whether conscious or unconscious. It comes to us in the food we eat, in water, in light from the Sun, but we have access to it in its most immediate form through air. The practice of meditation will help you to come to know for yourself the existence of this force in yourself and within all things.

Rhythmic breathing is a way of extracting more of this life-force and, by channelling it through the chakras, utilizing it more. By so doing the more vitality you will possess, the greater will become your sense of awareness, and the more effective will be your creativity.

Take a deep breath. Breathing in is an expression of the yin – the principle of receiving. Now bear in mind that what you are receiving is not just oxygen, but the life-force itself. Holding the breath is the unifying principle through taking in the life-force.

Now breathe out. Breathing out is an expression of the yang – and an outgoing projection of the will and intention. The pause before taking another breath is the neutralization – the pause before the cycle is repeated again.

This pattern of Raise – Hold – Release – Pause, is the same fluid motion, that powerful rhythm, that permeates Nature and is at the centre of all creativity. It is the rhythm of raising power within an energy-system, of controlling it and bringing it to its full potential, and then discharging it under the power of its own impetus.

By recognizing this pattern and by putting it into the same natural rhythm of the Earth – caused by the phases of the Moon, we harmonize with the natural energies of the planet. We become attuned with the Earth's energy-field. And we harmonize ourselves and become 'centred'.

That pattern and sequence has been discussed earlier when we examined the phases of the Moon – 11 days when the Moon is waxing, 3 days when it is full, 11 days when it is waning, and 4 days of the Dark Moon. This 11–3–11–4 pattern is the rhythm of the Earth's 'breathing'.

Try it now, just to get the hang of it. It is simply:

breathe in 1–2–3–4–5–6–7–8–9–10–11,

hold the breath 1–2–3

exhale 1–2–3–4–5–6–7–8–9–10–11,

pause 1–2–3–4.

As you establish this rhythm as part of your meditation practice, imagine as you take in each breath that the energy is being drawn up through your feet and filling your body, energizing every cell of your being as you hold the breath, and then giving away what you no longer need as you expel the air, and then pausing before the cycle is repeated.

Keep this routine going for three or four minutes, remembering that you are in your special mind-space. Then breathe normally.

4. Create the Vision

Visualization is the creation of a mental picture of an object or a situation. It is thinking in pictures rather than in words. It is seeing in the mind's eye an image of what is required, and so vividly that it takes on the appearance of an objective reality. Not everyone finds it easy. But it is a technique that cannot be worked at or striven for. It has to come gently and naturally.

In visualization you are making use of the power of your imagination, which is part of the creative energy of the universe, to create for you an image of what you want.

What now follows is a continuation of Creating the Power, for the power is activated by the use of creative visualization. The method I am now going to explain is a simple but effective way of developing the ability to visualize in meditation and to open up the power centres.

Having recharged the system through a few minutes rhythmic breathing, the next step is to imagine a glowing sphere of golden light just above the top of your head. With your eyes closed, 'see' it there hovering just above you like a miniature Sun. Now perform the rhythmic breathing sequence four times, sense the feeling of warmth descending into you.

Now imagine the ball of light has moved down to your throat area. Perform another four cycles of rhythmic breathing while it is there.

Let it move down to your chest and feel the energy from the golden sphere vitalizing your entire body as it rests there for four breathings.

Now let it descend to your navel and do four cycles of breathing while it is there. Then to your pelvic region for four breaths, and finally down to the area around your feet for four breaths.

Then, as you inhale, imagine to your count of eleven, that the energy from the sphere is rising up through you from your feet, up your legs to the base of your spine, then up inside your body to your neck and the top of your head. As you hold your breath to a count of three, see it like a jet coming out through the top of your head. Then, as you exhale, imagine it as a fountain of golden, shimmering light, descending all around the outside of your body and down to your feet. Then pause. Keep this image in your mind throughout a cycle of four breaths. Then return to normal breathing.

This will have begun to open up your energy centres and activate your imagination. You will not only feel deeply relaxed, but invigorated by the power of the life-force itself.

These four essential conditions should form the pattern of your meditation session to begin with and should be well established before you extend your meditation to include contemplation of any totem. After energizing the chakras you then merely visualize the totem – be it animal, plant or gemstone – that you wish to work with and then just observe: *look and listen*. Write down whatever thoughts and impressions come into your mind immediately you finish your meditation period.

So, set aside a period of twenty minutes to half an hour every day, if possible, but at least three or four times a week. The biggest difficulty is in setting up the routine in the first place and making the time for it. Once it is established and you have begun to experience the benefits, you will then treasure that period of your day.

Earth Medicine and the I Ching

THE ORIGIN OF THE *I CHING*, WHICH MEANS 'BOOK OF CHANGES', like the Medicine Wheel, is lost in pre-history, but we know it pre-dates the Confucianism and Taoism of the East and influenced them both.

In the West, the I Ching has become known as a means of predicting the future, like Sun astrology, but this is not one of its principal purposes, which is as an oracle, and that is not quite the same thing. An oracle is a means of measuring the quality of the moment and obtaining advice on its significance.

The Chinese revered the I Ching and approached it as if it were a very wise person, for if it is treated as if it were a person its replies are like personal replies.

The I Ching, the Medicine Wheel and Runes are designed according to a universal Law of Octaves, or cycles of eight. Like the DNA code, music theory, and computer binary notation, so the eight primary trigrams of the I Ching can be related to the Eight Directions of the Medicine Wheel. In Section Two, the eight primary trigrams have been assigned their appropriate places on the Earth Medicine Web and one of them is related to each of the twelve personality groupings.

A primary trigram represents a set of frequencies which are incorporated within the human energy-system. These impulses are indications of the way the individual personality is put together and can thus form the basis of a code or 'call sign' or 'function key' to access into the inner self and communicate with the Higher Self, 'divine' Self, True Self, or whatever name we choose to give it.

To complete the 'code', a question is asked and a further trigram obtained by the tossing of coins or the division of yarrow sticks, and this is built on top of the primary trigram to form a six-line symbol called a hexagram.

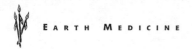

To the rational Western mind, a hexagram is thus formed in an entirely random manner using coins or yarrow sticks. But to the oriental mind and to the ancients, the pattern formed was not random at all, but a product of the moment. The use of coins or yarrow sticks was merely a mechanical device to tap a spiritual power which might be related to the subconscious mind. The hexagram or hexagrams arrived at when a question was put revealed to the individual's conscious mind how energies were moving towards a probable future, but one which could be changed by actions taken in the present.

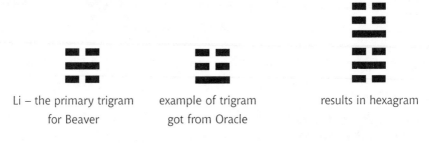

Li – the primary trigram   example of trigram   results in hexagram
for Beaver   got from Oracle

Consulting the Oracle is like stretching out time as if it were a rubber band. It is like looking down on a situation from a higher perspective and seeing a situation in a broader context. It can, perhaps, be likened to being in a car which is suddenly caught up in a traffic delay. From your seat behind the windscreen you cannot see beyond the vehicles immediately in front of you so you have no idea what lies further ahead. You can't tell how long you are going to be delayed, and you don't know the route well enough to know if there is a turn-off you can take to get round the source of delay. You can't see far enough ahead to know what is going on. You can only sit and wait and be the victim of circumstance.

But if you were looking out from the top window of a tall block of flats overlooking the road, you would be able to see the route you had followed to get where you were, and to see clear ahead for quite a long way. You would be able to see what was causing the traffic hold-up and, if it was an accident and emergency services were arriving, how long it was likely to be before traffic was able to get moving again. You would also be able to see where there were turn-offs and the best one to take to get you out of the line of traffic to make a quick detour of the situation.

Consulting the I Ching is like being able to switch your viewpoint from the window of car to a window at the top of a block of flats, or like plugging yourself in to advice from a traffic policeman viewing the scene overhead from a helicopter.

As we have seen, a trigram is a combination of three parallel solid or broken lines, there are only eight possible ways in which solid or broken lines can be combined in a trigram:

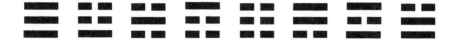

A trigram forms the lower and upper portions of a hexagram which is the full symbol needed to consult the oracle. From this joining together of two trigrams into a six-line hexagram, it is possible to develop sixty-four different combinations, or sixty-four different frequencies. And since one or more of the six lines can be a changing yin or a changing yang line the number of possible variations runs into many hundreds.

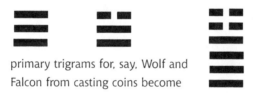

primary trigrams for, say, Wolf and Falcon from casting coins become

The coming together of two trigrams in this way indicates the interaction and dynamics not only of the subtle forces affecting the human condition, but of the interaction of the conscious and the subconscious within the individual.

Each hexagram forms a 'gateway' to show the way things are moving. Since movement enters the hexagram from the bottom, so the bottom line represents the beginning of a situation, and the movement flows upwards through its development and change to the top line, which indicates its likely outcome.

You obtain the trigram to build on top of the birth month trigram and thus into a hexagram by simply casting coins or by separating yarrow sticks and the use of the yang and yin principle I have already discussed in detail elsewhere in this book. I shall not describe the yarrow sticks method here since I want to keep the 'casting' as simple as possible. The use of yarrow sticks and the traditional Chinese way of 'working' the Oracle takes much longer than the coin method and is more ritualistic. A full explanation of this method is included in most books giving I Ching interpretations and you can make use of this method later if you so wish. I shall concentrate on the coin method which has the advantage of being both simple and effective.

The three coins you select for casting should be the same size, and small enough to be shaken within the cupped hands. Three newly minted pennies or cents are ideal, but any coins will do. Clean them first and leave them for a day or so in a salt water solution to cleanse them of grime and unwanted vibrations since they will have gone through many hands before they came into your possession, then put them aside for I Ching use only. The deck of I Ching Cards produced by the US Games Systems Inc., of New York, USA, comes complete with three special metal yin and yang coins with the numerical values also stamped on them. These are ideal, and the cards, too, are most helpful. In spite of the advice given in some books, it is not necessary to obtain old Chinese coins with square holes in them.

The three coins are shaken vigorously in the cupped hands and then simply dropped on to a flat surface.

A *head* is used represent *yin,* and counts as 2.

A *tail* is used represent *yang,* and counts as 3.

In casting the three coins and noting whether each comes up heads or tails – yin or yang – and adding up their values, you will come up with four possible totals from each throw of the coins:

6 (three heads).

7 (two heads and one tail).

8 (two tails and one head).

9 (three tails).

7 produces a *yang* and is represented by a *solid* line, thus: ▬▬

8 produces a *yin* and is represented by a broken line, thus: ▬ ▬

6 produces a *changing yin* – that is, a yin that is in the process of changing to its opposite, yang – and is represented as : ▬ x ▬

9 produces a *changing yang* – that is, a yang that is changing to yin and is represented as : ▬ o ▬

The first fall of the coins produces the bottom line of your new trigram, the second throw brings about the middle line, and the third throw produces the top line. You then locate your upper and lower trigrams on the Table of Hexagrams on page 302. It will give you the number of the relevant section of the Oracle to consult.

Before casting the coins, however, it is necessary to formulate your question. You must have it absolutely clear what it is you are seeking advice about. Take time to think your question through so that its wording is clear and precise. Write it down for the act of writing it will help to concentrate the mind.

When using I Ching in this way – that is, for the purpose of exploring the Medicine Wheel – questions should be limited to the kind that have a direct bearing on your own self-development. Remember, the primary trigram which forms the lower trigram of the hexagram, is attuned to the direction to which it is assigned and is therefore relevant to that direction and all things connected to it. It is being used as a 'key' to open up deeper chambers of the direction. So questions of a more general nature may require the building up of all six lines of a hexagram.

Avoid framing the questions that invite a Yes or No response. They are not questions, but indecisions. The Oracle is not for the purpose of telling you what to do and making decisions for you. For instance, 'What will be the effect of my taking this or that course of action?' should be asked rather than 'Should I do so-and-so?' Questions like, 'How can I best develop this or that quality?' 'What effect would (state the choice) have on my life?' and 'How am I likely to be affected by . . . ?' give an indication of the way questions should be framed.

After you have written the question down and examined it and are finally satisfied with it, try to see some sort of image of the question in your mind before you cast the coins. A face, perhaps, or a place, an object, an action, or a mannerism, connected with a quality being sought.

Once you have gained some experience and confidence in using the I Ching in this way, you may wish to seek guidance regarding a proposed 'move' to another segment of the Circle in order to acquire what it is you are seeking. You may be in some doubt as to where to go to first. In this case, don't put the question: 'Should I got to Beaver (or Snake, or whatever) to seek ways of strengthening this or that, or to aid me in whatever?' for this again invites only a Yes or No reply. Rather, ask the effect a 'move' to one direction is likely to have, and consider the answer you obtain. Then put the same question regarding another direction. Then compare the two responses, and weigh them up. The choice will be yours, but you will have obtained useful insights to enable you to consider the pros and cons.

The Table of Hexagrams chart on page 302 gives a number for each of the sixty-four hexagrams which is in accordance with their traditional order and the number given helps you to locate the interpretation of that symbol in any of the English translations or modernizations of the I Ching Oracle.

It is helpful to have more than one interpretation handy and to write down from each those phrases or sentences that 'ring a bell' in your mind. The Richard Bollinger translation *I Ching* (published originally by the Bollinger Foundation of New York in 1950 and by Routledge & Kegan Paul, London, in 1951, and of which there have been several subsequent reprints) is considered a classic, though the language in places may appear a little strange to the average Westerner. A more up-to-date interpretation is contained in *I Ching – a New Interpretation for Modern Times* by Sam Reifler, first published by Bantam Books, New York, in 1974. *The I Ching Workbook* by R. L. Wing, first published by Doubleday, New York, in 1974, is a very

UPPER TRIGRAM LOWER TRIGRAM	CH'IEN	CHEN	K'AN	KEN	K'UN	SUN	LI	TUI
CH'IEN	1	34	5	26	11	9	14	43
CHEN	25	51	3	27	24	42	21	17
K'AN	6	40	29	4	7	59	64	47
KEN	33	62	39	52	15	53	56	31
K'UN	12	16	8	23	2	20	35	45
SUN	44	32	48	18	46	57	50	28
LI	13	55	63	22	36	37	30	49
TUI	10	54	60	41	19	61	38	58

Table of the 64 Hexagrams

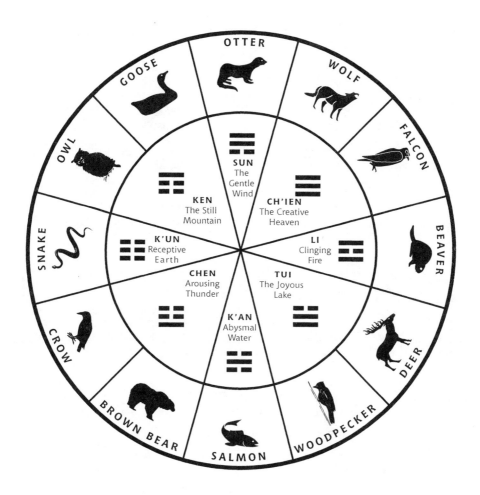

Figure 44. The Eight Primary Trigrams on the Earth Web

readable modernization, and was published in the United Kingdom by Aquarian Press in 1983.

If you have a 'Why?' question, like 'Why am I being faced with a repetition of (state the problem)?' or 'Why can't I make a success of (whatever it is)?', you should use what is called a nuclear hexagram.

A nuclear hexagram is built from the core – the nucleus – of the hexagram you have already obtained as a result of casting the coins after posing the question. It is constructed by taking the four middle lines of the hexagram – that is, lines 2, 3, 4 and 5 – and from these, the bottom lines (that is 2, 3 and 4) form the lower trigram of the new hexagram, and the

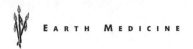
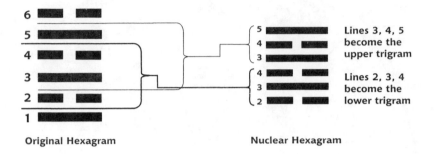

6

5

4

3

2

1

Original Hexagram

5   Lines 3, 4, 5
4   become the
3   upper trigram

4   Lines 2, 3, 4
3   become the
2   lower trigram

Nuclear Hexagram

Figure 45.

top three lines (3, 4 and 5) form the upper trigram. What we are doing is looking deeper into the heart of the hexagram to find the answer to a question Why? The Oracle is counsulted with the nuclear hexagram and not the original hexagram in dealing with 'Why?' questions.

Whatever method is used, the Oracle may not appear to answer your question directly. It may, on the other hand, appear to question your motives and urges. It may challenge you to examine a certain aspect more carefully. It might alert you to possible difficulties in pursuing a particular course of action. But it will never dictate what you should do, nor judge you, nor inflict burdens upon you.

Like a wise old sage and a respected elder who has experienced all the phases and ways of life, it will never tell you what to do, only enable you to see the issue more clearly and offer you the advice of a good friend.

Having used the I Ching in this way as part of your Earth Medicine workings, you may wish to extend it by making use of it in more general and traditional ways. Guidance is given in most books on the I Ching.

The Eight Fundamental Principles

EARTH MEDICINE HELPS US TO COME TO TERMS WITH HUMAN existence and to recognize that we are each part of the dynamic nature of the Earth environment in which we are experiencing consciousness in physical manifestation. Earth Medicine helps us to see ourselves as part of a greater Whole yet, paradoxically, to recognize that the whole is also within ourselves.

Earth Medicine is about character and the development and unfoldment of character because the character is our true 'face'. Everything else, including out physical looks, is but a 'mask'.

Earth Medicine is about extending the range of our perception and developing our inner senses so that we become more aware. Some people describe this extension of awareness as extrasensory perception. But this kind of perception is not 'extra' at all. It is not a question of developing extra senses. We can't obtain them from some external source of supply. We can't be awarded them by some educational establishment. We can't 'qualify' for them. We have them already. The trouble is that we haven't made use of them so they need to be awakened from their neglect. Earth Medicine helps that awakening.

Earth Medicine embraces the Eight Fundamental Principles of ancient wisdom:

1. The Principle of Mentalism

All is derived from spirit and fashioned by thought. Everything you see around you is solidified 'thought'. Every man-made object is the result of thought. Matter and energy are different expressions of spirit – one manifest, the other unmanifest.

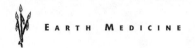
2. The Principle of Similarities

Whether manifest or unmanifest – everything is constructed of circles within spiralling circles and parallel spheres. So what is Within is mirrored Without. If one sequence is known on one Circle, another sequence of a similar type in a parallel sphere bears a proportional resemblance to it. In some philosophical schools of thought this is known as the Law of Correspondences.

3. The Principle of Rhythm and Vibration

Everything vibrates. Everything flows in and out and pulsates. The pendulum swing manifests in everything – the measure of the swing to the right is the measure of the swing to the left, and rhythm compensates. The atom is vibration. Thought is vibration. Change your mood or mental state and you change your personal vibration.

4. The Principle of Polarity

Everything is dual. Everything has polarity, and its pair of opposites. Opposites are identical in nature, but different in degree. Everything is yang or yin and has its masculine or feminine principle. Gender manifests on all planes. Conflicts are clashes of opposites. They can be resolved by bringing the opposites together to form a harmony, and Earth Medicine shows how this can be done. Otherwise, one opposite is repressed by the other and this dominance adds to the conflict.

5. The Principle of Connections

Everything in existence is an energy-system within a greater energy-system and comprises whirling and dancing groups in interpenetrating energy forms. Individual manifestations, whether human, animal, vegetable, mineral or celestial are thus connected like the strands of a spider's web.

6. The Principle of Cause and Effect

Every cause has an effect. Every effect has its cause. There are many planes of causation, and everything happens according to Law. Chance is the name of a law not yet recognized.

7. The Principle of Frequencies

Every individual is a set of personal frequencies. Everyone and everything has a personal vibratory pattern that is unique. Each pattern is different from all others, just as fingerprints are not matched by any other person. Earth Medicine provides knowledge of some of the frequencies that are shared with others so that they can be made use of to discover others. These frequencies are called totems.

8. The Principle of Self-Realization

You are not your body. You only use your body during Earth life because it is the most suitable vehicle for the Earth environment and for this lifetime.

You are not your mind. Your mind is used to think and to evaluate impressions reached through the physical senses and to discern physical reality.

You are the one who does the thinking. You are the one who chooses what to think. You are the Watcher Within. You can think, and with your thoughts you can create. You create through the power of the mind.

You are not matter at all, but spirit which is eternal and does not suffer death, only transformation.

The Sacred Laws

In addition to the Eight Fundamental Principles, there were also in being Sacred Laws which were universally applicable. They were sacred because they were the Laws of the very Being of the Great Spirit Itself and an expression of the will and mind of the One who created all with love and ensouled the universe with life.

According to American Indian cosmology and the ancient wisdom, when the Great Spirit created the material universe, the Cosmos was separated from Chaos by the Sacred Hoop or ring-pass-not. Within the Sacred Hoop was the universe which was organized in accordance with certain universal laws which became known as the Sacred Laws because they were the limitations the Great Spirit put on Itself and were the laws of our being also.

In the instant when the cosmos was separated from chaos, some chaos was trapped within the cocoon of the universe. Outside in the chaos were elements trying to get in and inside were elements of chaos seeking to get out, so the universe was permanently under stress.

According to this teaching of the ancient wisdom, about 20 per cent of all energy within the cocoon of the universe is random, so that although we can determine our position and create our own future through the choices we make, we cannot 'will' it all. There is a random or 'chance' factor in life which needs to be recognized. It was for this reason that in the American Indian culture and the tribal systems of ancient Europe, one was advised never to take life too seriously.

So, according to this teaching, though we can largely affect our own future we cannot determine it all. There is a factor at work in all our lives which cannot be controlled. Some religionists call it 'God's Will' and refer to accidents and catastrophes as 'Acts of God'. Of course, they are no such thing. They are not willed or caused by the Great Spirit, but they are allowed to happen by the Free Will of the Great Spirit and are brought about by the chaos factor which indirectly serves our own spiritual evolution and development and, indeed, serves to advance it.

Among the Sacred Laws, four were particularly stressed by American Indian shamans and by the shamans of the ancient cultures of Britain and Europe.

- Everything is an inseparable part of the One that is the Whole. Everything is completely and intimately linked with everything else.

- Everything is born of woman. All life comes into being through the feminine aspect, and therefore woman should be honoured and respected. The Earth is our Mother.

- Nothing must be done to hurt the children. This implied more than not causing harm. Future generations and the future of humanity, and therefore one's own future evolvement, rested in the children. To harm a child was therefore to harm one's own future.

- Maximum Efficiency with Minimum Effort. (This is the law of all energy in motion which follows the harmonic laws.)

There were other Sacred Laws but these four were at the heart of shamanistic teachings and of the wisdom of the ancients.

Conclusion

WHAT CAN WE CONCLUDE ABOUT OURSELVES FROM THIS STUDY of Earth Medicine? That we are Spirit Beings, individuated Spirit carried along elemental lines of energy and force and through one of the twelve vortices of expression and activity and into physical manifestation.

We are conscious beings – beings of Light. Not mortal beings with a spirit, but spirit beings with a body.

Our consciousness is the thinking and acting part of us that is looking out of a window on the world, and this is our individual perception point or the Circle of Life. Our consciousness enables the essence of our being – the Higher Self, the 'Spirit' or Soul Self – to comprehend the material realm as physical reality.

The Soul Self functions on different planes of existence contemporaneously, but our consciousness is usually aware only of physical reality because that is where the perception window is located at the present time. It is where our eyes are. It is where our 'I' is.

Establishing a link between the conscious, everyday self and the 'unconscious' Soul Self which transcends the carnal nature and the individual personality so that its impressions can be received by the brain, is true spirituality. True spirituality has nothing to do with religion or being 'religious'. It is a spiritual awareness based on practical experience that physical reality is not the only reality.

Physical reality has been described as 'ordinary' reality, for that is where the consciousness is 'ordinarily' for much of the time. But Earth Medicine has indicated that there is another reality, a reality of other dimensions that are not 'ordinary' and where the Soul Self may be contacted.

The Soul Self originates from a Source some have regarded as a divine Force or Supreme Being. Many people call it 'God', though their personification of that concept varies a great deal and is influenced by the culture and society into which they were born. To most people that divine Force, or Supreme Being, or 'God', is Something that is outside themselves. Someone who is outside the universe even. Some One 'up there' in a location called 'Heaven' that is beyond the stars, beyond the Here and Now, beyond even Space and Time, and to Whom we must somehow reach out, usually through an intermediary.

Earth Medicine and Medicine Wheel teachings indicate that humanity has got into its mess because for all too long it has been looking in the wrong place. It is the very act of regarding the Supreme Force as an external Personality outside the Creation that has actually insulated humanity from It and cut us off from our Source. Such action has short-circuited our design systems and we have blown a fuse which has prevented us from having access.

The 'unlearned' and 'ignorant' American Indian knew, as did the Masters of the Ancient Wisdom, that the Source was not *outside* but *inside* the Creation. Instead of looking outwards – 'up' there, to some place beyond reach, we should be looking inwards, *within* Creation itself, not outside it. Within ourselves, not outside ourselves. Nature shows us that, for the closer we get to anything in Nature, the more perfect it becomes.

We have to *experience* knowledge for ourselves in order for it to be acquired, and that is why Earth Medicine encourages us to find the time to *listen*. To listen to the Earth and what she has to say to us. To listen to the trees and the flowers, the birds, and the animals that run, or swim or crawl – they are all calling out and saying something to us, but humanity has deaf ears. Even the rocks and stones have things to tell us, for they, too, are manifestations of the Creative Source.

That is why Earth Medicine encourages us to *look*. To look *inward* so that we can better see outward. For Earth Medicine is a way of transformation – a changing of oneself in order that we might *be* one's self and when that happens the world is changed as we see it.

We have all of us spent so much time of our lives already in looking. Looking for love. Looking for security. Looking for satisfaction. Looking for fulfilment. Looking for opportunities. Looking for a good time. Looking for what? In a word – *happiness*.

But in our looking we have found that happiness is pretty elusive. It is not a territory that can be claimed. It is not something than can be owned. We can't hire it, borrow it, or steal it. We can't attract it to ourselves nor can we take it by force. Yet the world acts as if it can be obtained in one or more of these ways. We don't get it by seeking it for ourselves, but we can have it when we seek it for someone else. And that again is a key to finding it and experiencing it more permanently.

Happiness is a state without boundaries and without conditions because, quite simply, it is a condition of mind.

Earth Medicine is method of advancing our understanding of the universe in which we find ourselves, and of the Creative Source.

So many children and young people today are destructive, and vandalism is rife because they are being denied outlets for natural creativity. Everything is done for them. There is little opportunity for them to create for themselves. Their toys and playthings are manufactured. Without such off-the-shelf 'goodies' they are made to feel 'deprived' in a consumer-orientated society. Their energies are not used positively and creatively so they find expression negatively and destructively.

We all need to be creative because creativity is an expression of our Spirit. We all hanker to be creators. Yet the greatest creative work of all is the very life we have and which we are constantly fashioning, moment by moment. For every step we each take along life's journey is a moment of creation – the creation of our own future and our own destiny.

There is, then, a purpose in each of our lives that is something more than existence. There is more to our lives than earning a living and surrounding ourselves with whatever comforts take our fancy. Let us call it a 'higher' purpose since it transcends the purpose of making a living.

Our Soul Self knows what that purpose is, but we may no longer be conscious of it. Earth Medicine is a way of becoming so attuned that we can become aware of that purpose, for we shall never be truly satisfied until we are setting about fulfilling it. Whatever that purpose is specifically, it is in essence the same for each of us – expressing our own individual divine potential.

If, then, you want to bring out your potentials and you truly want to take control of your life and transform your circumstances, it is not enough just to have the knowledge that this book has to impart. You need understanding, and understanding cannot be learned. It just comes. It comes with movement and change, and Earth Medicine and the Medicine Way is about movement and change. But that means *using* the Web and travelling the Circle and living what it is you want to learn.

American Indians regarded every life as a Walk or Dance – a movement of creative energy around the Wheel of Life. The steps we take can tune us in to the rhythm of the planet and of the universe to form a choreography of harmony and beauty which is what the Soul Self intended.

Balance and harmony the Beauty Way was the spirit of the Native American peoples and of the Wise Ones of all races of old. And it is the spirit behind this book.

For centuries this ancient knowledge has lain hidden, guarded in part by the shamans and by the descendants of the 'wise ones' of many cultures to whom portions of it were entrusted. But for the most part it was withdrawn into the Great Unconscious but ready to surface again in the human soul through the inner planes when, in the fullness of time, conditions on Earth made it necessary as well as possible.

The time is now. The essence of the ancient wisdom is once again becoming manifest and available to all whose minds are open enough to receive it.

Walk in Beauty and we touch others and the Earth with the beauty of our innermost Self and bring healing to the planet.

The Great Spirit of the Redman

I am not separate from My Creation
Any more than your thoughts
Are separate from you.
I am not the Reality behind the world
But the Reality that is in it.
For I am in the world with you
In all your life
Wherever you are
Wherever you go
Wherever you look.
You can see Me in the Moon
And in the Stars
That bring forth light
Out of the darkness.
You can feel Me in the breeze
That kisses your cheek.
You can hear Me in the flowing waters
That refresh and renew.
The tiny seed that grows to a mighty oak
Contains My power
And the bud that blossoms forth in flower
Enfolds My fragrance.

I am with you now
In the ever-changing Present
That is true Eternity.
Closer than the breath
That brings your body life.
Closer than the thought
That springs within the mind
That ignorant men call finite
Closer than the beat
That keeps your heart in tune.
For I am to be found Nowhere
But where you are.
For I am the One that is All
And can be seen in all.
Anywhere.
Everywhere.
And I am the All that is One
In everyone.
So find Me now.
Touch Me now.
Feel Me now.
And love Me now.
Wherever you are.
Then you will Walk the Earth in Beauty.

Kenneth Meadows, 1987

Recommended Reading

Amerindians

The Teachings of Don Juan: A Yaqui Way of Knowledge. Carlos Castaneda, Penguin Books 1970–1986.

A Separate Reality. Carlos Castaneda, Penguin Books 1971-1986.

America B.C. Barry Fell, New York Times Book Co. 1976.

Book of the Hopi. Frank Waters, Penguin Books 1977.

Gospel of the Redman. Compiled by Ernest Thompson Seton and Julia M. Seton, Seton Village, Santa Fe, New Mexico 1966.

Lame Deer – Sioux Medicine Man. John Fire/Lame Deer and Richard Erdoes, Quartet Books, London W1P 1FD 1980.

Seven Arrows. Hyemeyohsts Storm, Ballantine Books, New York 1972.

The Medicine Wheel. Sun Bear and Wabun, Prentice Hall Inc., USA 1980.

Black Elks Speaks. As told to John G. Neihardt, Washington Square Press, USA 1959; University of Nebraska Press 1961; Sphere Books, London 1974.

Animals

Birds of Prey of the World. Eric Hoskings, Felham Books, London 1987.

The Psychic Power of Animals. Bill Schul, Coronet Books, Hodder Fawcett, London 1971.

Animal Speak. Ted Andrews, Llewellyn 1993.

The Aura

The Raiment of Light. David Tansley, Routledge & Kegan Paul, London 1984.

Chakras

Journey through the Chakras. Klansbernd Vollmar, Gateway Books, Bath, England 1987.

Colour

The Healing Power of Colour. Betty Wood, Aquarian Press, UK 1984.

I Ching

I Ching – a New Interpretation for Modern Times. Sam Reifler, Bantam Books, USA 1974.

I Ching – Book of Changes. The Richard Wilhelm translation. Routledge & Kegan Paul, London 1951–84.

I Ching Workbook. R. L. Wing, Aquarian Press UK and Doubleday & Co., New York 1983.

Tao of the I Ching. Jou, Tsung Hwa, Tai Chi Foundation, Taiwan 1984.

Meditation

Creative Meditation. Shakti Gawain, Bantam Books, USA 1982.

How to Meditate. Lawrence Le Shan, Turnstone Press, Wellingborough, England 1983.

Inner Guide to Meditation. Edwin C. Steinbrecher, Aquarian Press, UK 1982.

Meditation – a Foundation Course. Barry Long, Barry Long Centre, PO Box 106, London N6 5XS.

Meditator's Manual. Simon Court, Aquarian Press 1984.

Plants and Herbs

Book of Herbs. Kay N. Sanechi. Apple Press, London 1985.

Culpeper's Complete Herbal. J. Cleave & Son, Manchester, England 1826.

Handbook of Bach Flower Remedies. Philip M. Chancellor, C. W. Daniels, London 1973.

The Herb Book. John Lust, Bantam Books, USA 1983.

Reincarnation

Life After Life. Raymond A. Moody Jr., Bantam Books USA 1976.

Life Before Life. Helen Wambach, Bantam Books USA 1979.

The Case for Reincarnation. Joe Fisher, Grafton Books. London 1986.

The Evidence for Life After Death. Marton Ebon, New America Library Inc., New York 1977.

Rocks and Stones

Rocks and Minerals. Herbert S. Zim and Paul R. Shaffer, Golden Press, New York 1957.

The Magic of Precious Stones. Melice Uyldert, Turnstone Press, Wellingborough, Northants, UK 1981.

Shamanism

The Right Brain Experience. Marilee Zdenek, Corgi Books 1985

The Way of the Shaman. Michael Harner, Bantam Books USA 1982.

Shamanism. Compiled by Shirley Nicholson, Theosophical Publishing House, USA 1987.

Shamanism – the Foundations of Magic. Ward Rutherford, Aquarian Press 1986.

Voices from the Earth. Nicholas Wood, Godsfield Press Ltd, 2000.

Index

Kenneth Meadows appreciates receiving letters from readers, especially those relating to benefits gained from applying the principles explained in this book. He cannot, of course, guarantee to reply to every letter. Letters should be addressed to:

Kenneth Meadows
BM Box 8602
London WC1N 3XX
England